FIRST PLACE BIBLE STUDY

# CHOOSING
## *Thankfulness*

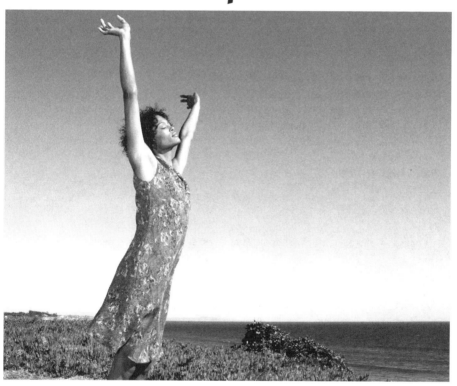

**Gospel Light**

FIRST PLACE™

**Gospel Light**

Gospel Light is a Christian publisher dedicated to serving the local church. We believe God's vision for Gospel Light is to provide church leaders with biblical, user-friendly materials that will help them evangelize, disciple and minister to children, youth and families.

It is our prayer that this Gospel Light resource will help you discover biblical truth for your own life and help you minister to others. May God richly bless you.

*For a free catalog of resources from Gospel Light, please contact your Christian supplier or contact us at 1-800-4-GOSPEL or www.gospellight.com.*

**PUBLISHING STAFF**
**William T. Greig,** Publisher • **Dr. Elmer L. Towns,** Senior Consulting Publisher • **Bayard Taylor, M.Div.,** Senior Editor, Biblical and Theological Issues • **Elizabeth Crews,** Contributing Writer

ISBN 0-8307-3818-5
© 2005 First Place
All rights reserved.
Printed in the U.S.A.

**Library of Congress Cataloging-in-Publication Data**
Choosing thankfulness.
     p. cm. — (First place Bible study ; 14)
  ISBN 0-8307-3818-5 (trade paper)
  1. Gratitude—Biblical teaching. 2. Bible—Study and teaching. I. Gospel Light Publications (Firm) II. Series.
  BS680.G74C46 2005
  220'.071—dc22

                  2005024245

Any omission of credits is unintentional. The publisher requests documentation for future printings.

---

**CAUTION**

The information contained in this book is intended to be solely informational and educational. It is assumed that the First Place participant will consult a medical or health professional before beginning this or any other weight-loss or physical fitness program.

---

# CONTENTS

# FOREWORD

My introduction to Bible study came when I joined First Place in March 1981. I had been attending church since I was a small child, but the extent of my study of the Bible had been reading my Sunday School quarterly on Saturday night. On Sunday morning, I would listen to my Sunday School teacher as she taught God's Word to me. During the worship service, I would listen to our pastor as he taught God's Word to me. Frankly, digging out the truths of the Bible for myself had never entered my mind.

Perhaps you are right where I was back in 1981. If so, you are in for a blessing you never dreamed possible. As you start studying the truths of the Bible for yourself through the First Place Bible studies, you will see God begin to open your understanding of His Word.

Almost every First Place member I have talked with about the program says, "The weight loss is wonderful, but the most important thing I have received from my association with First Place is learning to study God's Word." Bible study is one of the nine commitments of the First Place program. The First Place Bible studies are designed to be done on a daily basis. As you work through each day's study (which will take 15 to 20 minutes to complete), you will be discovering the deep truths of God's Word. A part of each week's study will also include a Bible memory verse for the week.

There are many in-depth Bible studies on the market. The First Place Bible studies are not designed for the purpose of in-depth study, but are designed to be used in conjunction with the other eight commitments of the program to bring balance into your life. Our desire is for each member to begin having a personal quiet time with God each day. This time alone with God should include a time of prayer, Bible reading and Bible study. Having a quiet time is a daily discipline that will bring the rich rewards of balance, which is something we all need.

God bless you as you begin this exciting journey toward a balanced life. God will richly bless your efforts to give Him first place in your life. Remember Matthew 6:33: "But seek first his kingdom and his righteousness, and all these things will be given to you as well."

*Carole Lewis*
First Place National Director

# INTRODUCTION

The First Place Bible studies were developed to be used in conjunction with the First Place weight-loss program. However, the studies could also be used by anyone who desires to learn more about God's Word and His will, with the added bonus of learning more about living a healthy lifestyle.

## A Balanced Life

First Place is a Christ-centered health program, emphasizing balance in the physical, mental, emotional and spiritual areas of life. The First Place program is meant to be a daily process. As we learn to keep Christ first in our lives, we will find that He is the One who satisfies our hunger and our every need.

God's Word contains guidelines for maintaining our physical well-being, equipping us mentally to make right choices, providing emotional stability to handle everyday circumstances as well as crisis situations and growing spiritually as we deepen our relationship with Him.

## The Nine Commitments

The First Place program has Nine Commitments that will help you draw closer to the Lord and aid you in establishing a solid, consistent and healthy Christian life. Each commitment is a necessary and important part of the goal of First Place to help you become healthier and stronger in all areas of your life—living the abundant life He has planned for each of us. To help you achieve growth in all four areas, First Place asks you to keep these Nine Commitments:

1. Attendance
2. Encouragement
3. Prayer
4. Bible reading
5. Scripture memory verse
6. Bible study
7. Live-It plan
8. Commitment Record
9. Exercise

# The Components

There are seven distinct components to this Bible study to aid you in bringing balance to your life. These components include the 10-week Bible study, two Wellness Worksheets, the leader's discussion guide, two weeks of menu plans, the Personal Weight Record, the 13 Commitment Records and the 10 Memory Verses.

## The Bible Study

Each week of each 10-week Bible study is divided into five daily assignments with Days 6 and 7 set aside for reflections on the week's lesson. The following guidelines will help make your study more enjoyable and profitable:

- Set aside 15 to 20 minutes each day to complete the daily assignment. It's best not to attempt to complete a week's worth of Bible study in one day.
- Pray before each day's study and ask God to give you understanding and a teachable heart.
- Keep in mind that the ultimate goal of Bible study is not only for knowledge but also for application and a changed life.
- First Place suggests using the *New International Version* of the Bible to complete the studies.
- Don't feel anxious if you can't seem to find the *correct* answer. Many times the Word will speak differently to different people, depending on where they are in their walk with God and the season of life they are experiencing.
- Be prepared to discuss with your fellow First Place members what you learned that week through your study.

## Wellness Worksheets

This study's Wellness Worksheets are interactive, will help you learn more about your style of expressing thankfulness, and will instruct you how to develop your own thankfulness journal to keep throughout this study.

## Leader's Discussion Guide

This discussion guide is provided to help the First Place leader guide a group through this Bible study. It provides information for the leader to prepare for each weekly group meeting.

## Menu Plans

The two-week menu plans were compiled from the *First Place Recipes* book and various fast food restaurants. Each menu is meant to simplify meal planning and include food exchanges. These meals are based on the MasterCook software that uses a database of over 6,000 food items and were prepared using United States Department of Agriculture (USDA) publications and information from food manufacturers.

## Personal Weight Record

The Personal Weight Record is for the member to use to keep a record of weight loss. After the weigh-in at each week's meeting, the member will record any loss or gain on the chart.

## Commitment Records

Thirteen Commitment Records (CRs) are provided in the back of this Bible study. For your convenience these have been printed on perforated paper so that you can easily remove them from the book and carry them with you through each week as you keep your First Place commitments. Directions for filling out the CRs precede those pages.

## Memory Verses

All 10 Memory Verses are listed on one perforated sheet and may be removed for memorization and review.

## Aerobic Workout DVD

The *Moving to the Word: Aerobic Workout* DVD features a 30-minute exercise routine with high- and low-impact aerobics led by certified fitness instructors. Use this DVD to strengthen your body and get closer to God's Word as you exercise to the sound of First Place Scripture Memory Music. You'll firm up your familiarity with God's Word as you develop a healthier body.

# THANKFUL FOR GOD'S ENDURING LOVE

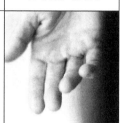

*MEMORY VERSE*
*Give thanks to the Lord, for he is good.*
*His love endures forever.*
*Psalm 136:1*

Have you ever wondered about God's will for you? All of us have times when we wonder just what God has planned for us. While Scripture does not give us specific directions as to which school to attend, where to live, which church to join or which car to purchase, God wants us to be inform-ed about what pleases Him. Speaking through the pages of Scripture, the Holy Spirit clearly reveals to us God's will regarding the most important decisions we will make.

One such passage is 1 Thessalonians 5:18, "Give thanks in all cir-cumstances, for this is God's will for you in Christ Jesus." Most of us read those words and quickly look for a different answer to our question about God's will! Yet our ability to thank God in the midst of adversity separates God's children from those yet in darkness.

Psalm 77:11-12 says, "I will remember the deeds of the LORD; yes, I will remember your miracles of long ago. I will meditate on all your works and consider all your mighty deeds." We are called to remember who God is and what He has done for us, confident that His kindness and love will continue throughout all generations. No matter how grim our present cir-cumstances, we can give thanks because our God is the same yesterday, today and forever.

## DAY ONE: *God, Our Reason for Praise*

This week's memory verse comes from Psalm 136. Throughout this Psalm, every example of God's enduring love is followed by the phrase "His love endures forever." This Psalm was meant to be read responsively; the choir sang about the good things God had done for His people, and the congregation affirmed His enduring love by their response. Imagine what a magnificent sound must have filled the courts as the choir sang and the people reaffirmed their faith in the God of Abraham, Isaac and Jacob! By studying this Psalm, we too can be assured of God's enduring love.

Psalm 136 can be divided into five sections, each of which tells a different truth about the faithful love of our Lord. Today we will focus on verses 1 through 3; but before answering questions specific to these verses, take time to read the entire Psalm. Try to picture the glorious scene inside the temple. Pretend you are in the congregation, shouting "His love endures forever" as you praise the God of gods and Lord of lords.

In verses 1 and 3, we see two variations of the word "lord": "Lord" and "LORD." In Hebrew (the original language), these are not the same word. Lord refers to God's authority over His subjects; LORD is the covenant name for God.

➤ Turn to Exodus 6:6-8 to find out the significance of the word "LORD." What did you discover?

➤ What else does Psalm 136:1 tell us about this LORD we are thanking?

➤ Read Romans 8:28 and James 1:16-17 to learn more about God's goodness. According to these verses, how does God use His goodness for *our* good?

➤ Psalm 136:2-3 tells us another important truth about the LORD. What do these verses affirm?

➤ In the following space, list five specific and personal ways that the God of gods and Lord of lords has been good to you:

1.

2.

3.

4.

5.

Conclude today's lesson by reading each of the statements you wrote in answer to the previous question followed by the words of Psalm 136:1, "Give thanks to the LORD, for he is good. His love endures forever." If possible, speak out loud as you recount God's goodness in your life.

Sovereign LORD, You are good and Your love endures forever. Thank You for allowing me to be among the joyful throng called to sing Your praises throughout eternity.

You are the God of gods and the Lord of lords. "I will meditate on all your works and consider all your mighty deeds," which manifest Your kind love to those who are sealed with Your name (Psalm 77:12).

# DAY TWO: *God, Our Creator*

"In the beginning, God created the heavens and the earth" (Genesis 1:1).

Psalm 136:4-9 tells us about some specific aspects of God's good creation. Prayerfully read these verses, and then list what aspect of creation each verse recalls.

Verse 5

Verse 6

Verse 7

Verse 8

Verse 9

➤ According to verse 4, God is the only One who does great wonders. What happens when we attribute miracles to someone other than God alone?

➤ What allowed God to make the heavens (v. 5)?

➤ After reading Job 38:1-18, summarize God's understanding of the world He created.

Pause for a moment and ponder, *If God were to ask me why I question His wisdom and stubbornly refuse to acknowledge Him as my creator, how would I try to explain my stubborn resistance to His revealed will for my life?*

Psalm 136:7-9 tells us that God made the sun, moon and stars to govern each day and night.

➤ What similarities do you see between Psalm 136:7-9 and Psalm 19:1-6?

In his letter to the Romans, the apostle Paul described those who did not acknowledge God or give Him thanks, even though God made Himself visible to them.

➤ According to Romans 1:18-20, how has God made Himself known to all humankind?

Write a prayer in the following space, acknowledging God's power and giving Him praise for the wonders of His creation. Affirm ways that creation reveals God's unfailing love and thank Him for knowing you intimately.

 "O LORD, our Lord, how majestic is your name in all the earth! You have set your glory above the heavens" (Psalm 8:1). I am without excuse if I do not acknowledge You and give You thanks for Your marvelous deeds.

By Your understanding the earth was created. Lord, I will trust You instead of questioning Your wisdom by leaning on my own understanding (see Proverbs 3:5).

# DAY THREE: *The Lord, Our Deliverer*

Verses 10 through 15 of Psalm 136 speak of God's unfailing love as He delivered His people from bondage and cruel oppression. Read these six verses that speak of God's mighty acts on behalf of His oppressed people.

➤ On Day 1, we examined Exodus 6:6-8. Reread that passage and then explain why Psalm 136:10-15 shows evidence of a LORD who keeps His covenant promises to His people.

➤ Compare Exodus 6:6 with Psalm 136:12. How did God deliver His people?

God's mighty hand and outstretched arm symbolize His might and power as He goes forth to accomplish His purposes. In sharp contrast to God's mighty hand that guarantees victory, Scripture describes another hand—a hand of oppression and destruction. The cruel bondage the children of Israel suffered at the hand of Pharaoh and his taskmasters is symbolic of our slavery to the bondage and oppression of sin, especially as it manifests itself in addiction. Before coming to First Place, we too were under a hand of oppression and destruction because of our addiction to food.

➤ Describe your addiction and how it kept you enslaved. Avoid generalizations. List specific ways you were imprisoned by your relationship with food.

God manifests His faithfulness and love to us by using the First Place program to free us from our bondage and oppression. If you were writing a praise psalm, what statements would you make about the ways God's mighty hand and outstretched arm have freed you from slavery?

→ List five specific ways your Deliverer has helped free you from the cruel bondage of addiction. List your participation in First Place as one of the ways.

1.

2.

3.

4.

5.

Now repeat the exercise from Day 1 by reading these five statements out loud, followed by the words of Psalm 136:1, "Give thanks to the LORD, for he is good. His love endures forever."

Almighty God, with an outstretched arm and mighty acts You have freed me from the yoke of slavery. I will give You thanks, for Your love does endure forever (see Exodus 6:6).

Sovereign Lord, You are the same yesterday, today and forever (see Hebrews 13:8). Just as You freed the children of Israel from Pharaoh, You deliver me from my oppression.

# DAY FOUR: *The Lord, Our Protector*

God does not deliver us and then leave us to fight our battles alone! Once He had delivered the children of Israel from the hand of their oppressor, Pharaoh, He led them through the desert and gave them victory over new enemies. Psalm 36:16-22 recounts how God destroyed enemy forces as He led His people to the Promised Land. Reread those verses now and find strength and hope in those words. God, who never changes, does the same thing for His children today. Not only has He freed you from oppression, He will shepherd you until you reach green pastures and calm waters (see Psalm 23:2).

≫ Read the following passages. Who fought for the Israelites? Write your findings beside each verse.

Exodus 14:14

Deuteronomy 1:30

Deuteronomy 3:22

Joshua 23:10

Nehemiah 4:20

≫ The same God who fought for the Israelites fights for us as well. Look up the following New Testament passages. Who is the source of our victory? Once again, record your findings beside each verse.

Romans 8:37

1 Corinthians 15:57

2 Corinthians 2:14

1 John 5:4

You do not fight spiritual battles in your own strength and power. Jesus Christ fights your battles and guarantees your victory as you travel toward the Promised Land.

➢ List five specific obstacles you have overcome through your faith in Jesus Christ, the One who overcame the world and broke sin's reigning power.

1.

2.

3.

4.

5.

As you did on Days 1 and 3, read each of the five statements and follow each one with the words of this week's memory verse.

Sovereign Lord, just as You fought for the children of Israel, You give us victory through Christ, who loves us and gave Himself for us.

I love You, O Lord, my strength. You are worthy of all praise. When I call to You in my distress, I am saved from my enemies (see Psalm 18:1,3).

## DAY FIVE: *The Lord, Our Provider*

As the Israelites traveled through the desert on their way to the Promised Land, they faced many enemies who inhabited the hostile land they crossed, but they also faced an even greater enemy because they forgot to remember God's mighty deeds.

Shortly after crossing the Red Sea, Moses sang a beautiful song of praise to God. Turn to Exodus 15:1-18 and read the song Moses and the Israelites sang to God on that glorious day.

Exodus 14:31 tells us what happened to the Israelites as a result of their powerful deliverance. Look up this passage and fill in the blanks:

> And when the Israelites _____ the great _____
> of the _____ displayed against the Egyptians, the people
> _____ the _____ and put their _____ in
> him and in _____ his servant.

Now read Exodus 15:22-24 to see what happened just three days after the people rejoiced in God's deliverance and put their trust in Him.

➣ What happened to the confidence the Israelites had expressed three days earlier? What was the cause of their distress?

Lack of water was not the only peril the children of Israel faced as they traversed the desert.

➣ Read Exodus 16:1-3. What was the cause of the people's distress in this passage?

➣ When faced with the fear of hunger, what happened to their memory of Egypt?

Memories of food made the Israelites long to go back to the oppression from which God had saved them! How much like those frightened people we are. We cried out to God in our misery and pain and He delivered us. Yet at the first thought of hunger, we remember all the food we had when we were still in bondage.

≫ In His mercy, God didn't send the Israelites back to Egypt for their complaining. According to Exodus 16:11-16, what did He do instead?

≫ How has God shown you mercy when you longed for your former lifestyle?

≫ Psalm 136:25 reminds us of another reason to thank God. What is that reason?

≫ What does each of the following verses tell us about God's provisions?

Psalm 23:1

Psalm 90:14

Psalm 103:5

Psalm 145:16

How can you apply these truths to your involvement in the First Place program?

➳ Write a prayer of thanksgiving to the God who satisfies your desires with good things.

 Gracious God, how quickly I forget what You have done for me and begin to grumble and complain. Forgive me, Lord, for doubting that You will satisfy my desires with good things.

LORD, You are my shepherd. I shall not lack anything (see Psalm 23:1).

## DAY SIX: *Reflections*

"Euphoric recall" is a term used to describe a selective memory process that causes recovering addicts to recall how good they felt when they were using their drug of choice—but to somehow forget how foolishly they behaved and the dire consequences of their behavior. Because of euphoric recall, memories of "how it was" are always filtered through distorted perceptions. Remembering how good the high felt, in the absence of recalling the painful consequences, keeps addicts from fully realizing the unmanageability of their disease and the depth of their addiction. As a result, euphoric recall limits addicts' abilities to truly admit their powerlessness and their total dependence on God to deliver them from their addiction.

Euphoric recall isn't limited to recovering addicts. Recall what you learned in Day 5 about the Israelites' selective memory. They remembered the good food they had in Egypt and that it was at no cost—when in reality they paid a very high price for that food: bondage and slavery. They remembered the meat, cucumbers, melons, leeks, onions and garlic, but not the cruel taskmasters who oppressed and mistreated them. They remembered the pleasure and forgot about the price and the pain.

Many of us in First Place also suffer from euphoric recall. We remember the delicacies we ate prior to coming to this program. We recall how good they tasted. We talk about how we were able to do things in the past that don't fit into our new First Place lifestyle. But we forget the high price we paid for the privilege of indulging in self-destructive behavior. How quickly we remember the pleasure; how quickly we forget the pain our undisciplined eating caused us. Somehow we don't recall the disordered lifestyle that kept us continually off balance and in despair.

Today, rather than looking back at what we had when we were in bondage to our cravings, let us remember the benefits of living a life that is pleasing to God. Instead of wailing about not being able to indulge our appetites, let us remember the life we now enjoy because we are putting God first in all things and reaping His abundant blessings. God gives us all good things for our enjoyment. Who are we to question the wisdom and understanding of the One who created the world through His unlimited understanding and mighty power?

One way to combat euphoric recall is to keep a record of just how bad it really was. As part of today's reflections, devote a page in your spiritual journal to this project. Tell yourself the truth about what it was like to be enslaved to a powerful addiction to food. Mark this page so you can find it quickly the next time you find yourself remembering "how good it was" prior to joining First Place. At the end of your writing, thank God for His providential care as His mighty hand and outstretched arm delivered you from the bondage that characterized your former way of life.

 Almighty God, I am part of Your good creation. Help me to never destroy what You have made for the sake of food (see Romans 14:20).

Sovereign Lord, I will meditate on Your faithfulness and love instead of recalling the pleasures of sin that kept me enslaved and in cruel bondage.

Thank You, God of heaven, for all You have done for me. You remembered my low estate and saved me from all my enemies. You provide for all my needs today and throughout eternity, for Your love endures forever (see Psalm 136:23-26).

# DAY SEVEN: *Reflections*

Living lives characterized by thankfulness does not come naturally to our human condition. If it were inherently part of our being, Scripture would not have to admonish us to be thankful in all circumstances, to rejoice always and to be content with God's generous provisions. Left to our human inclinations, we would be filled with envy, strife and irritability rather than with abundant thankfulness. Only by the Holy Spirit's power within us can we be obedient to God's command to be thankful people.

The choice to be thankful is both a one-time commitment and an ongoing decision. The process begins when we make the choice to be thankful rather than follow our natural tendencies to find fault and complain. After this initial commitment to a lifestyle of thankfulness, we will be faced with situations each day that will test our resolve. In these moments, we can either decide to give God thanks and to trust that He is working all things together for our good, or we can fall back into self-pity and begin questioning God's faithfulness.

If we are to develop a lifestyle of thankfulness, we must undergo a paradigm shift. We must transform the way we view the world around us and the circumstances we face, and we must consciously look for the positive and reject the temptation to dwell on the negative. Recall from the introduction to Day 1 how the psalmist was able to turn all the happenings of his life into an opportunity to thank God. To refresh your memory, write the words of Psalm 77:11-12 below.

How was the psalmist able to remember all the good things that God had done for His people? Someone had taken the time to write down what God had done so that His mighty deeds could be recounted! So it is with us. In order to meditate on God's enduring love, we need to keep a record of the good things God does in us and around us by keeping a written record of His kind love. We need to become mindful of the ways He delivers us, fights for us and provides for us. One of the easiest ways to foster an attitude of thankfulness is to create a separate place to record those simple, everyday things for which we are grateful.

Wellness Worksheet One will explain how you can create and maintain a thankfulness journal—a daily record of the good things God has done for you and others. In order to get the maximum benefit from this Bible study and to develop a lifestyle of thankfulness, faithfully keep a thankfulness journal for the next nine weeks. Spend some time today reading Wellness Worksheet One and creating a thankfulness journal so that you too can begin recording God's mighty deeds on your behalf.

 You are the Lord my God, who brought me out of bondage. I will open my mouth wide, trusting You to fill it with good things (see Psalm 81:10).

O Lord, I will meditate on the great works You have performed in my life and I will consider all Your mighty deeds (see Psalm 77:11-12).

Today I will give You thanks, O Lord, for You are good and Your love endures forever (see Psalm 136:1).

# Group Prayer Requests   Today's Date:_____

| Name | Request | Results |
|------|---------|---------|
|      |         |         |
|      |         |         |
|      |         |         |
|      |         |         |
|      |         |         |
|      |         |         |
|      |         |         |
|      |         |         |
|      |         |         |
|      |         |         |
|      |         |         |
|      |         |         |
|      |         |         |
|      |         |         |

# THANKFUL FOR GOD'S STRENGTH

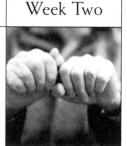

MEMORY VERSE

*For the Mighty One has done great
things for me—holy is his name.*
Luke 1:49

As soon as we begin looking at the exhortation to give thanks in all circumstances, it becomes obvious that this is not something we can do in our own strength and power. Left to our natural inclinations, we too would grumble and complain, doubt God's provision and accuse Him of withholding good from us, just as the Israelites did.

From where exactly do we get the ability to give thanks? This week we will examine God's Word to answer the question, "Where does my help come from?" (Psalm 121:1). With the psalmist, we will discover, "My help comes from the LORD, the Maker of heaven and earth" (v. 2).

## DAY ONE: *The Source of Our Strength*

God's name and God's character are one and the same. It is impossible to separate God's name from His attributes, for they are synonymous. God often reveals parts of His nature to His children by the names He uses to describe Himself.

➤ Read Genesis 17:1 and 35:11. By what name did God refer to Himself when speaking with Abraham and Jacob?

The Hebrew word for Almighty, *El Shaddai,* literally means "complete, perfect or having integrity."[1]

➣ What does the meaning of El Shaddai tell you about God's power and might?

Psalm 91 vividly describes what it means to dwell in the shadow of the Almighty. Take a few moments to read this psalm now.

➣ In verses 14 through 16, God makes eight promises to those who love Him. List these promises below.

1.

2.

3.

4.

5.

6.

7.

8.

➣ Which of these benefits do you need to take advantage of today by placing yourself in the shadow of the Almighty? Why?

What do you need to eliminate from your life so that you can place yourself in His shadow and receive the benefits He has promised to those who love Him?

Are you willing to take the action steps necessary to place yourself under His mighty hand? If so, list one step toward that goal that you will do today, and then begin to take action!

El Shaddai, You are my refuge and my fortress. I trust in You (see Psalm 91:2).

Jesus, You told Your disciples that they showed their love for You by their obedience. Help me to obey Your command to give thanks in all circumstances, knowing that thanksgiving honors You as the Mighty One who sustains and comforts me in trouble.

## DAY TWO: *Songs of Thanksgiving*

Our memory verse this week comes from the song of thanksgiving Mary sang after the angel Gabriel told her she would give birth to the long-expected Messiah.

Looking at Mary's circumstances from the world's eyes, she had very little reason to be thankful. She was a poor, unwed mother, expecting a child who had not been conceived by her soon-to-be husband. Had Joseph not been a kind, compassionate man who believed God's message, he could have had her stoned. Yet in the middle of seemingly unfortunate circumstances, Mary sang the praises of the Mighty One.

Turn to Luke 1:46-55 and read Mary's words.

>> What do you find most striking about Mary's song? Describe your thoughts as you read this passage.

Now turn to 1 Samuel 2:1-10 and read the song of thanksgiving another mother, Hannah, sang. Like Mary, from the world's perspective Hannah had little reason to rejoice. Her precious son, the one for whom she had begged God, had to stay in Shiloh while she went home to Ramah. Those of us who have children and grandchildren know how difficult it is to leave a child on the first day of school. But Hannah was leaving her son for good with an aging priest in a town far from her home.

>> How are Mary and Hannah's circumstances alike?

>> What similarities do you see in Mary's and Hannah's words?

>> How would you react if you were in either of their circumstances? Give careful thought to your answer.

Given the similarities in Mary's and Hannah's reactions and word choices, it is likely that both women were reciting psalms they had learned from memory. Interestingly, these women would not have had access to Bibles because the scrolls were only available to the priests. Even if Bibles had been available, most women in biblical times could not read. People memorized Scripture by reciting it from childhood, and devout Jews knew much of the book of Psalms by heart.

How do Mary's and Hannah's responses emphasize the importance of memorizing Scripture?

How can the memory verse commitment of First Place help you to give thanks in all circumstances?

In addition to each week's memory verse, you might consider memorizing other songs of thanksgiving, like psalms or other passages of Scripture, so that you can recite words of thanksgiving in the midst of adversity. List one such passage below and make it part of your daily prayer this week.

My heart rejoices in You, O LORD. There is no other Rock like You (see 1 Samuel 2:1-2).

My soul glorifies You, O Lord, and my spirit rejoices because You are God, my Savior (see Luke 1:46-47).

## DAY THREE: *Music at Midnight*

Mary and Hannah aren't the only examples from Scripture of people who sang songs of thanksgiving in the midst of adversity. Today we will open our Bibles to the book of Acts, where we find the account of Paul and Silas's night spent in a dark jail cell in Philippi. Turn to Acts 16:22-34 and read this account before answering the following questions.

➣ Verse 22 tells us that the mob was hostile and that Paul and Silas were the objects of their anger. What is the first thing the city magistrates did in an attempt to remedy the situation?

➣ What happened next (v. 23)?

➣ Upon receiving orders to watch Paul and Silas carefully, what did the jailer do (v. 24)?

➣ Pretend you are a television reporter on assignment in Philippi. Describe the events of the story to this point as if you were giving a report to a worldwide audience. Include your observations and describe how you think Paul and Silas felt after all that had happened to them that day.

➣ How would you have responded if you were bruised and bleeding and locked in a dark, heavily guarded jail cell?

✎ According to verse 25, how did Paul and Silas respond?

"[They were] _____ and _____ hymns
to _____."

Verse 25 tells us that the other prisoners were listening to Paul and Silas's songs of praise, even though it was the middle of the night.

✎ How can your prayers and hymns to God in the midst of adversity affect people around you who might otherwise never be exposed to the gospel?

✎ Paul and Silas's midnight music also got someone else's attention. Who came to Paul and Silas's aid as they were praying and singing hymns?

✎ Continue your on-location report by giving a vivid account of the events described in verses 26 through 34.

Because Paul and Silas gave thanks in all circumstances, this story has a joyful ending. Complete the following sentence based on the information in verse 34.

The jailor's entire _____ was filled with _____ because they had _____ to _____ in God.

➤ Drawing on the events described in today's lesson, summarize the connection between giving thanks in all circumstances and being a powerful witness for Jesus Christ.

Gracious and Sovereign Lord, thank You for calling me to be a witness to Your goodness and grace through my ability to give thanks in all circumstances.

Almighty God, I will trust in Your unfailing love; my heart will rejoice in Your salvation. I will sing to You, my Lord and my King, for You have been good to me (see Psalm 13:5-6).

## DAY FOUR: *Strength in Weakness*

This week we have looked at several men and women who gave God thanks and praise in the midst of seemingly impossible circumstances. Scripture speaks of many more saints who sang songs of thanksgiving from pits of despair. Desperate circumstances are often opportunities for God to reveal His mighty power to save.

The apostle Paul often found himself in desperate circumstances. We are told that Paul had a "thorn in the flesh" that he asked God to take away—not once . . . not twice . . . but *three* times.

➤ Turn to 2 Corinthians 12:7-10. Write the Lord's answer to Paul's request, found in verse 9, below.

Whenever we see the word "therefore" in Scripture, we need to stop and ask, "What is it there for?" The verses before the conjunction tie the thoughts together.

Continuing in verse 9, Paul said:

*"Therefore* I will _____ all the more _____ about
my _____ so that _____ power
may rest on me" (emphasis added).

➣ Based on the information given before we see "therefore," why was
Paul committed to boasting gladly about his weaknesses?

➣ According to verse 10, why could Paul delight in weaknesses, in
insults, in hardships, in persecutions and in difficulties?

➣ Give an example from your own life of a weakness or adversity you
have repeatedly asked God to remove (e.g., a physical limitation, a
mental or emotional handicap).

Do you feel as though God has not heard and answered your prayers
because He has not taken away this source of distress? If so, how do
you express your frustration?

How might your attitude and response change if you were to see your
weakness as an opportunity for God's power to be made perfect in
you?

➤ Turn back a few chapters to 2 Corinthians 4:7. In New Testament times, clay pots were fragile, dispensable and ordinary. Why did Paul say that we have the treasure of the gospel in "jars of clay"?

How can you use your weakness to display God's strength through the First Place program?

➤ Write a prayer of thanksgiving to God for the weakness that brought you to the First Place program.

 Thank You, Lord, for the light of the gospel and for Your Spirit, who displays Your all-surpassing power in my life (see 2 Corinthians 4:7).

Almighty God, I will glory in my weaknesses because they allow Christ's strength to rest on me (see 2 Corinthians 12:9).

# DAY FIVE: *Confidence in God*

David wrote many of his psalms while he was being chased by his enemies, yet they often contain beautiful songs of thanksgiving. Through reading the book of Psalms, we learn how to bring our laments to God in an honoring way and are encouraged to give thanks in all circumstances.

David didn't hide his emotions from God. He expressed the whole range of human emotion. He laughed and danced when life looked up, but he also cried out when he was angry, frustrated and afraid. Many of us can learn from David's honesty.

What prevented David's passionate displays of feelings—often in the form of questioning complaints—from being offensive to God? What distinguished them from distrust? In the midst of his questions and complaints, David expressed confidence in God as the source of his help. Often this change in tone is signaled by the little words "but" or "yet"; other times it takes the form of praise in the middle of sorrow-filled words.

Today we will look at some psalms of lament to see how the psalmists brought their complaints and their confidence before God in songs of thanksgiving.

➤ Prayerfully read the following psalms. Look for the pivotal point when complaint turns to affirmation of confidence in God. In the space next to each psalm, write the cause of the psalmist's distress and identify the pivotal word that changes his song of lament to a song of confident praise.

Psalm 13

Psalm 54

Psalm 130

The psalmists often wove complaint and confidence throughout their laments, and we can do the same in our prayers.

Think of a current situation in your life that is causing you pain. Perhaps you want to list the complaints on a separate piece of paper before you begin to write your lament. Now turn your questions and complaints into a psalm of praise. After you have expressed your distress, affirm your confidence in God and His ability to save you from your situation. Reflect back on His tender mercies in the past. End your psalm with a strong affirmation of your trust in God. For privacy and to allow more room to express your passionate feelings and your steadfast trust in God's faithful love, you may wish to do this exercise in your prayer journal rather than in the space provided.

O Lord, I will put my hope in You, for with You is unfailing love and full redemption (see Psalm 130:7).

"Hear my prayer, O God; listen to the words of my mouth" (Psalm 54:2).

# DAY SIX: *Reflections*

Business letters often end with some version of the request "Thank you in advance for your prompt attention to this matter." However, what we consider standard business etiquette is often sorely lacking in our most intimate conversations with God. When was the last time you thanked God in advance for what you asked to receive? While we thank others for their time, attention and consideration of our requests, we come to God like demanding children. Even before we properly address Him as Father and tell Him how important He is to us, we begin to recite our laundry list of expectations.

Jesus followed a different pattern. He often looked up and thanked His Father, not for granting His request, but for hearing Him. Having thanked His Father for His time, attention and consideration, Jesus then acted as though His request had already been granted. Instead of hemming and hawing and saying "I don't know if this is Your will," Jesus thanked God and then took action. Jesus' example teaches us that thanking God in advance for something we have requested is a high form of prayer. Such an anticipatory prayer implies confidence that we are His children and that He will give us our heart's desire when we take the time to tell Him what we need.

Your First Place prayer journal is an excellent place to thank God in advance for hearing your requests. We are not strangers who can only be heard by a prearranged conference call. We are always welcome in God's presence. When you write your prayers in a prayer journal rather than on random sheets of loose paper, the pages in the journal become a sacred written record of your most intimate conversations with your Lord. However, even though we take the time to thank God in advance for hearing our heartfelt cries, it is good to reread those precious pages often so that we can thank Him again for the wonderful way He has taken our requests and brought them to pass in His perfect time and all-knowing way.

Take time today to use your First Place prayer journal to thank your Father in advance for hearing your prayers. Then use what you have learned this week to present your questions and complaints to God. Conclude by affirming your faith in His Mighty power and your willingness to allow His strength to cover your weaknesses.

 Almighty God, I will praise Your name in song and glorify You with thanksgiving (see Psalm 69:30).

You are the Mighty One who has done great things for me, and I am filled with joy (see Psalm 126:3).

O God, You have surely listened and heard my voice in prayer. Thank You for not rejecting my words or withholding Your love from me (see Psalm 66:19-20).

# DAY SEVEN: *Reflections*

For most of us in First Place, the adage "the crack in the jar lets the light in" has new meaning. We have discovered that our life has a flaw—a flaw that has caused us untold misery and despair. No matter how well we seemed to get the rest of our life together, getting our eating habits under control somehow eluded us. Certainly we could follow diets for a short time. Most of us were even successful at losing some weight, but soon we found ourselves falling back into old habits. We were up, down, and back up again as we rode the diet roller coaster that passed normal so fast that most of us forgot what normal really was. As a result of our diet failures, we felt cracked beyond repair. Some of us even considered this excess weight to be the "cross" that Jesus had asked us to bear.

We are now discovering that what we once considered a curse is actually an opportunity for God's healing light to shine in and through our lives. The crack in the jar that we once considered to be a flaw has been transformed into an opening—an opening for God's truth and light to fill our beings and a window for the Light that we carry inside of us to shine through us. As we remain faithful to the First Place commitments, our flaws become fissures of grace. Not only do we radiate His love, but we also become a beacon of hope to those still struggling under the oppression of out-of-control eating. Today we no longer need to blame our genes, our family, our friends, ourselves or our God for our flaws. Now we can see God displaying His power in our lives—and see our flaws as opportunities for His power to be displayed in and through us for His glory, honor and praise.

Spend some time right now meditating on this week's memory verse. Write the verse at the top of a journal page and then make a list of all the great things the Mighty One has done for you. Perhaps you would like to end your quiet time by singing or reciting the words to the time-honored hymn "Holy, Holy, Holy" or another song that speaks of the great things God has done for His chosen people.

O Lord, You are the Mighty One, yet You treat me with gentleness and compassion. I can be weak in Your presence because I know You will never do anything to betray my trust in You.

Maker of heaven and Earth, You are my refuge and my fortress. Keep me safe as I trust in Your provision (see Psalm 91:2).

You are the Mighty One who has done great things for me—Holy is Your name (see Luke 1:49).

Note

1. *The International Inductive Study Bible*, "Note on Genesis 17:1" (Eugene, OR: Harvest House, 1993), p. 26.

# GROUP PRAYER REQUESTS  TODAY'S DATE:_____

| NAME | REQUEST | RESULTS |
|------|---------|---------|
|      |         |         |
|      |         |         |
|      |         |         |
|      |         |         |
|      |         |         |
|      |         |         |
|      |         |         |
|      |         |         |
|      |         |         |
|      |         |         |
|      |         |         |
|      |         |         |
|      |         |         |
|      |         |         |
|      |         |         |

# THANKFUL FOR GOD'S COMPASSIONATE CARE

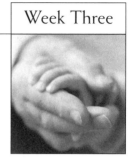

### MEMORY VERSE

*He brought me out into a spacious place;*
*he rescued me because he delighted in me.*
Psalm 18:19

Of all the visual images God uses to describe Himself in Scripture, perhaps the one that best portrays the Father's compassionate care of His
children is the analogy of the Good Shepherd tenderly leading His flock.
When we feel small and helpless, the Good Shepherd takes us in His arms
and holds us close to His heart. When we stray from the flock and find
ourselves entangled in a thicket of sin, He rescues us. When we are lost
and confused, He comes looking for us. When fierce predators threaten
our safety, He is our strong protector. When we are wounded and in pain,
He binds up our wounds, places us on His broad shoulders, and carries us
until we are strong enough to walk on our own again.

➤ Before starting this week's study, write a description of your favorite
image of the Good Shepherd and explain why this mental picture is
so meaningful to you.

## DAY ONE: *Thankful We Are His Sheep*

In the first line of Psalm 23, David—both a shepherd as well as a grateful sheep in His Master's pasture—declared, "The LORD is my shepherd, I
shall not be in want." This oft-quoted statement contains both a boast and

a profound display of trust. David's words reflect an inner contentment that marks a lifestyle of thankfulness.

Turn to Ezekiel 34 and prayerfully read verses 1 through 10 before answering the following questions.

➤ Obviously, these verses do not describe the Good Shepherd! What words or phrases came to your mind as you read Ezekiel 34:1-10?

➤ List five ways God described the negligent shepherds of Israel who took care of themselves while the sheep that were entrusted to their care perished.

1.

2.

3.

4.

5.

➤ List five specific things that happened to the unfortunate sheep who found themselves in the care of the self-serving shepherds.

1.

2.

3.

4.



5.



When we examine a shepherd's relationship with his sheep, we notice that the welfare of the flock is completely dependent on the compassionate care of the shepherd. The shepherd determines the fate of his flock! If the shepherd is diligent and faithful, the sheep will prosper; if he is careless and abusive, the sheep will wander aimlessly and suffer great harm.

Close today's lesson by writing a prayer of thankfulness that you are not left to wander over the mountains and become food for savage beasts. With David, affirm that the Lord is your Shepherd and that because of His compassionate care, you can lie down in green pastures and live in peace.

 Lord Almighty, today I kneel in humble gratitude, thanking You for not leaving me in despair and neglect. Because You are my Shepherd, I shall not want. Help me, LORD, to see Your compassionate care as I dwell contentedly in Your pasture, today and always.

Shepherd of my soul, thank You for loving me and for carrying me back to Your fold when I was lost and afraid.


## DAY TWO: *Thankful He Saw My Plight and Rescued Me*

Abuse and neglect are two words we hear often today, but praise God that He cares about those who are subjected to cruel treatment and comes to their rescue. Today we will resume our study of Ezekiel 34; but before you begin today's lesson, spend a moment or two remembering the plight of the sheep we learned about yesterday.

Now read Ezekiel 34:11-16.

≫ In verse 11, God describes Himself as the Sovereign _____.

≫ Refer back to week one, Day 1. What is the significance of the name "Lord"? What does this Lord promise to do for His people?

For review, write a brief description of what the Almighty LORD did for His people when they were slaves in Egypt.

In today's passage, we see the sovereign LORD once again noticing the plight of His chosen people and intervening to rescue them. In contrast to the mighty deeds and spectacular miracles God used to deliver Israel from bondage during the Exodus, Ezekiel shows us a different facet of God's love and care.

≫ What words would you use to describe the Shepherd's actions on behalf of His mistreated and abused sheep as recounted in Ezekiel 34:11-16?

≫ In the space below, write Ezekiel 34:16 as it appears in your Bible. Then go back and circle the action verbs that describe what God has resolved to do for His mistreated sheep.

✎ Which one of those six specific acts do you need God, the faithful Shepherd of your soul, to carry out on your behalf today?

A wonderful way to remember the meaning of the word "intimacy" is to sound it out as "in-to-me-see." God, who desires an intimate relationship with you, sees into your deepest being. He knows exactly what you need and will come to your rescue when you cry out to Him.

Write a prayer-filled letter to God, telling Him about any abuse or neglect that you are presently experiencing. You can either use the space below or, for privacy, write this prayer in your spiritual journal.

The same God who sees your heart wants you to see into His caring, compassionate heart and discover just how very much He loves you! God invites you to intimately know Him.

✎ What attribute of God have you seen in today's lesson that was hidden from you in the past?

Thank the Lord for revealing Himself to you today in this new way.

 Compassionate and caring God, You are my LORD. Thank You for rescuing me when I was lost and in peril. Without Your love, I would have been eternally lost and left to wander aimlessly in a barren land.

Tender Shepherd, when Your people suffer, You suffer with them. Thank You for caring about my inner hurts and for inviting me into an intimate relationship with You. Thank You for allowing me to know You in new ways today so that I can continue to sing Your praises throughout eternity.

## DAY THREE: *Thankful for Green Pastures*

Not only does our caring, compassionate God care about how His sheep are treated by the shepherds charged with their care, God also cares about how the sheep treat one another and the pasture they inhabit.

Returning to Ezekiel 34, read verses 17 through 24. In this passage, God talks about two other forms of abuse and neglect.

⟶ What two other kinds of mistreatment angered God?

God had every right to be upset with these sheep; they fouled up the good pasture God gave them to enjoy and they bullied and harmed one another. Sheep who are not well cared for take out their anger and frustration on the environment and on the other sheep who share the land with them.

⟶ What were God's specific complaints against the sheep and goats who made the pasture uninhabitable through careless behavior (v. 18)?

⟶ Can you picture the deplorable condition of the pasture? Now contrast that image with the Good Shepherd's pasture as described in Psalm 23.

What could have prevented the disaster in the neglectful shepherds' field?

Ultimately, the condition of the field is the responsibility of the shepherd. Had the shepherd properly managed and disciplined the sheep instead of neglecting them and leaving them to their own devices, this pollution would not have occurred. A well-managed herd of sheep replenishes and restores the condition of the fields. Sheep under the care of an uncaring shepherd can do untold destruction to the very land they depend on for survival.

➤ Turn to John 10:10. In this passage, Jesus was also talking about the Good Shepherd and His sheep. What did Jesus say the thief comes to do?

➤ Regardless of what form the thief takes, who is the real villain who works to destroy the Good Shepherd's flock? (Check your answer by reading Revelation 12:9.)

➤ By connecting Jesus' words in John 10:10 with our study of Ezekiel 34:17-24, what can you learn about those who do not care about the condition of the world that God has given them to inhabit and enjoy?

➤ Write this week's memory verse in the space below. Underline the reason God rescues His flock from the clutches of the evil one and gives them pleasant pastures in which to dwell.

➤ Spend a moment relishing the thought that God delights in you, and then write an affirmation that expresses your gratitude for His caring compassion.

God of the heavens and the earth, thank You for giving me spacious, pleasant surroundings because You delight in me.

Tender and loving Shepherd, today I am thankful that You give me healthy food to eat and clear, clean water to drink. Help me to protect and preserve Your good creation as a sign of my love and gratitude.

## DAY FOUR: *Thankful for Caring Companions*

When we examined Ezekiel 34:17-24, we identified two things that were going on in the flock that displeased the Lord: (1) His sheep were carelessly polluting their environment and spoiling His good creation; and (2) There was strife and contention within the flock. The stronger sheep were bullying the weaker sheep and vying for power and control.

Yesterday we saw that the ultimate responsibility for the condition of the pasture belonged to the shepherds. Lack of proper husbandry had allowed the flock to foul the field they inhabited. Today, as we continue our study of Ezekiel 34:17-24, we will examine the second problem: The sheep were not treating one another with kindness and compassion.

The lack of harmony within the flock was also the product of careless shepherding. Without loving discipline and proper guidance, the flock was not self-controlled or respectful, especially toward the weak and disadvantaged.

Not only does the Good Shepherd embrace the responsibility He has for the sheep that are entrusted to his care, His care and compassion also extend to the way the sheep in His flock treat one another.

➳ Turn in your Bible to Galatians 5:13-15. As you read these verses, what thoughts come to mind?

    . What does verse 14 admonish God's people to do?

➳ Describe the similarities between the destructive behavior described in verse 15 and the state of the mismanaged flock we read about in Ezekiel 34.

➳ Based on Galatians 5:16-18,22-26, what would have remedied all the problems the flock experienced?

➳ Now read Ezekiel 34:25-31. What promises did God make to His faithful flock in this passage?

How are these promises similar to the promise we studied in Exodus 6:6-8?

➺ According to John 10:11, Who is the Good Shepherd that God sent to fulfill the promise He made in Ezekiel 34 to care for His flock?

Lord Jesus Christ, You are the Good Shepherd, sent by God to save me from my sins so that I can live in harmony with my spiritual brothers and sisters.

Thank You, Jesus, for Your care and compassion that rescued me from a life of self-destruction, abuse and sin.

## DAY FIVE: *Thankful for Application*

The Bible becomes more real to us when we are able to take passages, like the ones we have been studying in Ezekiel 34, and apply them to situations in our daily lives. As we seek to personalize Ezekiel 34 today, we will see why this chapter is so pertinent to the First Place program.

On Day 1 of this week, we looked at a group of people who had abused and neglected God's sheep in order to promote their own well-being. Prior to coming to First Place, we may have put ourselves under the care of diet gurus who did the same thing—individuals who took advantage of our plight in their quest for financial gain.

➺ Recall a time when following the regimen of a fad diet left you weak, injured or wandering in the darkness of depression. What was God's caring, compassionate solution to your despair?

Stop for a moment and spend some time thanking your Shepherd for leading you to the green pasture of First Place.

> Based on your study of Ezekiel 34, how do you think God feels about individuals and companies that prey on the misfortune and despair of others, especially those who are weak and desperate?

What can you do to help liberate those who are still the victims of fad-diet marketing schemes?

Many of us belonged to diet support groups before we came to First Place. These groups may have been full of competition and rivalry rather than love, encouragement and support.

> Have you ever been in a diet group in which you were humiliated and demeaned because others were losing weight more quickly than you were? If so, describe how that experience made you feel.

Part of developing a lifestyle of thankfulness is learning to encourage others who may be weak and struggling. Take the time right now to write a note to someone in your First Place group who could benefit from an extra measure of encouragement.

Those of us who have experienced God's compassionate care are called to pass that care and compassion on to others. Mismanaged sheep leave a wake of destruction behind them. Goodness and mercy are the legacy of the righteous. Resolve today to be an ambassador for Christ by spreading a pathway of blessing everywhere you go.

 Gracious God, thank You for leading me to the First Place program and for putting me in a group of caring Christians who can reflect Your love to me because You have met their needs.

Loving and merciful Father, today I am thankful that You have called me to be part of the triumphal procession of Christ. By Your grace, I can be the fragrance of the knowledge of Christ as I march on my way to my heavenly home (see 2 Corinthians 2:14).

## DAY SIX: *Reflections*

Those caught in the throes of addiction leave a path of destruction in their wake that often resembles a hurricane's devastation. Broken relationships, lost jobs, irate friends, financial chaos—the damage, like the addiction, permeates every aspect of the addict's life. For those caught in the addiction of compulsive overeating, another telltale sign follows in our wake: a trail of junk-food wrappers and food crumbs!

On this day of reflection, spend some time remembering what your environment used to look like. Picture your favorite TV chair. Was it full of crumbs? Were there candy bar wrappers stuffed in the pockets and creases? Were there food stains on the carpet near where you sat? What about your car? Was it full of fast-food cartons and food residue? Were there ketchup stains on the upholstery? Did it smell like a garbage can? Once you have a vivid image in your mind, draw a picture that depicts the mess you left behind when you came to the First Place program.

In addition to a trail of wrappers and crumbs, there were other signs of our disease. Our eating habits were not the only thing out of control! In what other ways did compulsive overeating affect your environment? Did excess weight keep you from maintaining your yard and cleaning your home? Was your clothing slovenly or your appearance disheveled? Perhaps in your depression and despair you even neglected basic personal hygiene.

➽ Make an honest assessment of the damage your food addiction caused in other areas of your life.

Thanks to God's caring compassion, that dire picture has changed. Now that we are on the road to healthy living, we no longer leave trails of garbage behind us! Our lives are no longer out of control. We now leave trails of blessings in our wake that line the path of Christ's disciples. Not only do goodness and kindness come to us, they flow through us. Our cup, overflowing with God's love, spills over to everyone He puts in our path.

Write a prayer in your journal, thanking God for allowing you to break free from the destructive bondage of addiction so that you can experience the freedom found only in Christ Jesus. The Good Shepherd loves you and invites you to care for others as a reflection of that love.

LORD, You have done great things for me and I am filled with joy (see Psalm 126:3).

Gracious God, thank You for blessing me so that I can be a blessing to others and spread the fragrance of life everywhere I go (see 2 Corinthians 2:16).

Praise to You, Lord Jesus Christ. I am no longer imprisoned by my destructive ways. I can walk in the newness of life because You care for me!

## DAY SEVEN: *Reflections*

Providence can be described as provision for the future through benevolent guidance in the present. Though it is connected to the word "provide," it means much more than simple provision. Providence describes God's mighty hand and outstretched arm going out ahead of His people and preparing the way. Providence describes a God who orchestrates everything together to accomplish His purposes.

If you have ever arranged a large gathering, you know how difficult it is to coordinate the people, the food and the entertainment in some kind of orderly fashion! Now multiply that effort to include all the events taking place all over the world on any given day. Can you imagine trying to keep all the details in order? And yet, even this illustration does not adequately portray God's providence. He providentially weaves innumerable circumstances together to bring good to His children.

Because of our First Place testimonies, we are living examples of God's providence. Stop for a moment and recall all the events that brought you to the First Place program. Now picture the others in your First Place group and the providence that brought them to the First Place program. Consider how the First Place program came to your church. Now expand your vision to include all the First Place participants and leaders worldwide.

Spend time today thanking God for His providence—the marvelous way He orchestrates all things together for the good of those who love Him. When we meditate on God's providential care in our lives, we too can declare, "Give thanks to the LORD, for he is good. His love endures forever" (Psalm 136:1).

≫ Write this week's memory verse in the space below. By now, you should know it from memory!

≫ Using the words of this verse, describe why your Good Shepherd leads and guides you by providentially orchestrating all your circumstances.

≫ Now, list one action step you can take today to begin cooperating with God's process of masterfully weaving all things together for His glory and your good—which are always one and the same!

O Lord, all Your ways are loving and faithful. Remember me according to Your love, O Lord, for You are good (see Psalm 25:7,10).

Lord God, I will give You thanks, for You are good and Your love endures forever (see Psalm 106:1).

Sovereign Lord, You are the Potter and I am the clay. I am shaped by Your masterful hands as You mold me into the image of Christ (see Jeremiah 18:6)

# GROUP PRAYER REQUESTS   TODAY'S DATE:_____

| NAME | REQUEST | RESULTS |
|------|---------|---------|
|      |         |         |
|      |         |         |
|      |         |         |
|      |         |         |
|      |         |         |
|      |         |         |
|      |         |         |
|      |         |         |
|      |         |         |
|      |         |         |
|      |         |         |
|      |         |         |
|      |         |         |
|      |         |         |
|      |         |         |

# THANKFUL FOR GOD'S GUIDANCE

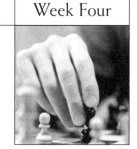

## MEMORY VERSE

*The Counselor, the Holy Spirit, whom the Father
will send in my name, will teach you all things and
will remind you of everything I have said to you.*
John 14:26

Last week, we studied Ezekiel's prophecy that foretold a day when God
Himself would shepherd His people. Several centuries later, that prophecy
was fulfilled. This week, as we continue to develop a lifestyle of thankfulness, we will turn our attention to the ways the Good Shepherd leads His
flock and patiently guides His precious ones into all truth.

## DAY ONE: *Thankful He Calls Me by Name*

Read John 10:1-18 out loud so that you can hear yourself proclaiming God's
Word. When you have finished reading, answer the following questions:

➤ According to verse 11, who is the Good Shepherd? How did He show
His love for His sheep?

➤ Read John 1:29. How is Jesus described in this verse?

In laying down His life for His sheep, Jesus Christ, the Good
Shepherd, also became one of the flock.

John 10:7-8 reveals more truth about Jesus. What do these verses teach about our Savior?

How does this truth compare with Jesus' words in John 14:6?

According to John 10:3, how does the Good Shepherd get His stubborn sheep out of the pen?

In your Bible, underline the phrase, "He calls his own sheep *by name* and leads them out" (emphasis added). Reflect on this passage as you go about your day. Bask in the truth that God knows you by name! In Scripture, a person's name is synonymous with the very essence of his or her being. God knows all about you and calls you anyway! Perhaps you would like to write that amazing fact in your thankfulness journal right now.

John 10:3,16 tells us that the Good Shepherd's sheep *listen* to His voice. Part of the prayer commitment of First Place includes taking the time to do just that. In your quiet time today, thank God for knowing you intimately and for calling you by name. Then listen for His voice and allow Him to lead and guide you throughout your day.

Lord Jesus Christ, You are the way, the truth and the life. Thank You for loving me enough to lay down Your life for me (see John 10:11; 14:6).

Loving Father, how precious are Your thoughts toward me! My name is even engraved on the palms of Your hands (see Isaiah 49:16).

# DAY TWO: *Thankful Jesus Came Looking for Me*

While Jesus was on Earth, He faithfully led His disciples and sought out the lost sheep of Israel. Those of us who attended Sunday School as children learned a story about one such lost sheep—a "wee little man" named Zacchaeus. Today we will look at his story through adult eyes.

Turn to Luke 19:1-10 and read about Zacchaeus's conversion.

≫ How does Luke describe Zacchaeus at the beginning of the story (v. 2)?

What else do we learn about Zacchaeus (v. 3)?

≫ Although Zacchaeus wanted to see Jesus, there were some obstacles that could have kept him from that desire, including his financial success. What did Zacchaeus do to overcome his limitations (v. 4)?

≫ What obstacles—physical, mental or emotional—have kept you from actively seeking Jesus (e.g., social prejudice, compulsive busyness, preoccupation with money, anxiety over the future)?

What have you done to creatively overcome your challenges?

➤ In your own words, what happened to Zacchaeus because he was willing to do whatever it took to see Jesus (vv. 5-6)?

➤ What did the people who were observing this miracle-in-the-making have to say about what was happening (v. 7)?

➤ When you first welcomed Jesus into your life, were there people who felt you were not worthy of Jesus' time and attention? Perhaps the committee in your head taunted you with comments like, *How could Jesus possibly care about an awful sinner like me?* If so, how did this opposition make you feel?

➤ What did Zacchaeus do to quiet the critics (v. 8)?

➤ What things have you been willing to give up so that others can see how important a relationship with Jesus is to you? Giving up your disordered relationship with food through participation in First Place could certainly be part of this list.

➤ How does the story of Zacchaeus reinforce the truth found in Hebrews 11:6?

⇛ How has the First Place program helped you to earnestly seek Jesus?

End today's lesson with a prayer of thankfulness. Rejoice over the salvation that has come to you because Jesus came to seek and save the lost.

Lord Jesus, You came to seek and save the lost (see Luke 19:10). Thank You for finding me and coming to stay in my heart, even though I was a sinner.

While I was still a sinner, Christ died for me. Thank You, gracious Father, for sending Your Son so that I can be part of Your family (see Romans 5:8).

## DAY THREE: *Thankful for an Invitation to Follow*

Yesterday we saw an example of a man who was richly rewarded for doing what it took to be in a right relationship with God. Of course, not all conversions are that dramatic. Jesus works in every believer's life in His perfect way and in His perfect time. Just as we are unique, our calls from Jesus are also unique.

Today we will turn our attention to four simple fishermen who heard the words "Follow Me!" Open your Bible to the first chapter of the Gospel of Mark and read verses 16-20.

⇛ What was Jesus doing that paralleled the story we read yesterday about Zacchaeus (v. 16)?

Jesus is always on the move, willing to meet us right where we are. We don't need to be at church or on a spiritual retreat to be in His presence. Andrew and Simon were going about their daily routine as fishermen.

≫ What did Jesus say to Andrew and Simon, and how did He make His words relevant to them (v. 17)?

≫ Although Andrew and Simon knew what it meant to be fishermen by trade, do you think they had any idea what Jesus meant by the phrase "fishers of men"? Why or why not?

Have you ever wondered exactly what Jesus was asking of you when you heard Him say, "Follow me"? How did your uncertainty influence your decision to respond, or not to respond, to His call?

≫ What did Simon and Andrew have to do in order to follow Jesus (v. 18)?

What did that act imply?

≫ Verses 19 and 20 tell a similar story about two other brothers. What did James and John give up in order to follow Jesus?

What might fishing nets and the family businesses represent in your own life?

Are you willing to give up the source of your security and significance and walk into the unknown in order to follow Jesus? Some of the things you might have to give up include thoughts, prejudices, resentments and personal ambitions. Following Jesus always means giving up every self-destructive behavior such as compulsive overeating, which abuses your body, mind, emotions and spirit.

Talk to Jesus about the fear this question raises in your heart and why you are reluctant to drop your nets and follow Him. Record your conversation with Jesus in your prayer journal. Remember, He already knows what you are thinking before you write one word on the page, so you have no reason not to be 100 percent honest with Jesus—and with yourself.

➤ How does letting go of the things that keep you from following Jesus relate to Matthew 6:33, the foundational verse of the First Place program?

How is letting go connected to living a lifestyle of thankfulness?

➤ We easily forget that in order to be led, we must agree to follow. What one thing can you do today to begin the process of letting go so that you can make a wholehearted commitment to follow Jesus and put Him first in all things?

 God of peace, You brought back from the dead my Lord Jesus, my great Shepherd. Equip me with everything good for doing Your will. Work in me what is pleasing to You, through Jesus Christ, to whom belongs all glory forever and ever (see Hebrews 13:20-21). Amen.

# DAY FOUR: *Thankful I Was Not Abandoned*

After three short years of ministry, the time came for Jesus to complete His mission and go back to the Father. Jesus knew He would have to die a painful death in order to fulfill the Scriptures. Yet even in His agony, Jesus was concerned for His disciples. In John 14—16, Jesus comforted His disciples and told them that they would not be left alone.

➤ What did Jesus promise His disciples in John 14:18?




Earlier this week, we saw that Jesus Christ was the fulfillment of God's promise to send a Shepherd to care for His sheep. The coming of the Holy Spirit is also the fulfillment of a promise God made to His covenant people.

➤ Look up Deuteronomy 31:6 and Joshua 1:5. What promise did the LORD repeat in both verses?




Have you ever taken the time to thank God for fulfilling His promise to never leave you or forsake you? You have not been orphaned or left alone. That is reason for rejoicing!

➤ What does God's promise to never leave you or forsake you mean to you with regard to your participation in the First Place program?




➤ Write this week's memory verse from memory.

➢ What do you need the Holy Spirit to teach you today about putting Christ first in all things? List at least one specific thing you need to know so that you can better follow the Nine Commitments of First Place.

➢ According to James 1:5, what does God do when we ask Him for wisdom?

What does He *not* do in response to our request?

Never be afraid to ask the Holy Spirit for wisdom and guidance. That is one of His divine purposes. He came to guide you into all truth and to teach you everything you need to know in order to lead a life that pleases God (see John 16:13). He will never chide you for asking a "dumb" question!

Add to your thankfulness journal the wonderful assurance that you have not been abandoned or left to face your problems alone. Spend some time in prayer, thanking God for the gift of His Holy Spirit.

Father, forgive me for those times I fear that You have forsaken me and have left me to go back to my old way of life. You have promised to never leave me alone. Today I will remember Your great and precious promises so that I can escape the corruption of the world (see 2 Peter 1:4).

Sovereign Lord, I can be content with what I have because You promise to never leave me or forsake me (see Hebrews 13:5).

# DAY FIVE: *Thankful for the Spirit of Truth*

Before His death and resurrection, Jesus introduced His disciples to the Holy Spirit. Jesus told them it was to their advantage that the Spirit take His place. As long as Jesus was on Earth in human form, His presence was limited by time and space. Because Jesus' physical body did not allow Him to be in two places at one time, He could not be present with all of His disciples all of the time. However, Jesus told His disciples that once He was with them in *Spirit*, He would always be with each of them, every moment of every day. They would never again be separated by time or space.

➤ Read Ephesians 3:14-19, and then complete the following sentence:

God _____ us with His _____, so that Christ may _____ in our hearts through _____.

How is this faith the same as the faith the disciples exhibited when they dropped their nets to follow Jesus?

➤ Do you have faith that the Holy Spirit lives in your heart, giving you the power to do everything God calls you to do, such as following the Nine Commitments of First Place? If so, describe how you know that the Holy Spirit lives in you.

➤ In order to better understand how the Spirit works in your life, read the following verses:

John 14:26

John 16:8-11

John 16:12-14

≫ John 16:8 says that the Spirit convicts us of sin. What sin in your life—anything that separates you from God—might the Spirit want you to address? Are you listening to His gentle voice or are you ignoring His council?

≫ Though being convicted of sin feels extremely uncomfortable, why is it a reason to be thankful?

≫ Recite this week's memory verse, John 14:26, aloud. What truth do you need to be reminded of right now so that you can begin cooperating with the Spirit as He guides you into all truth?

Thank You, Father, for not giving me "a spirit of timidity, but a spirit of power, of love and of self-discipline" (2 Timothy 1:7).

My Lord and my God, with the help of the Holy Spirit who lives in me, I will guard what You have entrusted to me (see 2 Timothy 1:14).

# DAY SIX: *Reflections*

In the Gospel of John, we are introduced to the ministry of the Holy Spirit, who dwells by faith in the heart of all believers. Just before He was crucified, Jesus told His disciples, "I will ask the Father, and he will give you another Counselor to be with you forever" (John 14:16). Jesus could no longer be with His followers in physical form, but He would not leave His frightened, confused disciples to fend for themselves. The *New International Version* translates the name "Jesus" that is used to describe the Holy Spirit in John 14:16 as "Counselor." However, when we limit the ministry of the Spirit to the confines of that name, we miss out on much of Jesus' intent. Of course, the Spirit does give comfort, counsel and help, but He does much more than that. In the original language, Jesus referred to the Holy Spirit as *paracletos*, which literally means "one who is called in." Paracletos is used to describe:

- A witness who is called in to give evidence for the defense
- A lawyer who is called in to plead the case of an accused man
- A friend who is called in to give counsel and advice
- A doctor who is called in to give help and healing
- A person with dynamic power who is called in to encourage those who are discouraged and afraid[1]

"Paracletos" is actually an ancient warrior term. Greek soldiers went into battle in pairs so that when the enemy attacked, they could draw together back-to-back, covering each other's blind side. A paracletos was called in to enable a soldier to cope with any situation life threw his way. In modern-day verbiage, the Holy Spirit has got our backs in battle!

Only through the power of the Holy Spirit dwelling within us are we able to keep the Nine Commitments of the First Place program. Without the Spirit of Truth, we cannot benefit from this program designed to bring health, balance and restoration to our bodies, minds, emotions and spirits. Review the Nine Commitments and choose the commitment with which you most need your Paracletos's assistance. Write Him a letter in your prayer journal asking Him for help. Finish your letter by thanking Him for going into battle with you and for covering your blind side. He's got your back!

Father, I am so thankful that the Spirit intercedes for me when I don't know how to pray. Thank You for sending Him to be with me forever (see John 14:16).

Lord, thank You for sending the Holy Spirit to teach, guide and encourage me so that I can follow the Nine Commitments of First Place more faithfully.

## DAY SEVEN: *Reflections*

For the past two days, we have been learning about all the great things the Holy Spirit brings to the lives of those who have accepted Jesus Christ as their Savior and Lord. At the very millisecond we invite Jesus to dwell in our hearts through faith, the Holy Spirit takes up residence and begins to do His transforming work in us.

There is yet another aspect of the Holy Spirit's ministry that we dare not overlook: The Spirit intercedes for us in prayer. The apostle Paul put it this way, "We do not know what we ought to pray for, but the Spirit himself intercedes for us with groans that words cannot express" (Romans 8:26). The following simple story illustrates the apostle Paul's words:

> It seemed that the copy machine in the church office was not working properly. It was Friday afternoon, and Sunday's bulletin was still a work in progress. In desperation, the pastor, who was not mechanically minded, called the repair shop to see if they could tell him what the problem was and how to fix it. But to his dismay, he quickly discovered that he didn't even know how to describe what was broken. He didn't know the names of the parts or what was specifically wrong. All he knew was that it was Friday afternoon, Sunday's bulletin still had to be run, and the copy machine wouldn't work. Sensing the urgency of the situation, the repair shop agreed to send out a technician right away. Once the technician arrived at the church office, he made a thorough examination of the broken copier. Then the tech called the repair shop. Unlike the pastor, however, he knew just how to describe what was wrong. He used words the pastor didn't understand, but the expert at the shop understood precisely what the technician was saying and gave the tech clear instructions on how to

remedy the problem. Soon the copier was repaired, the bulletin had been run and the pastor was praising God that someone had been called in who could solve the problem quickly and efficiently. His need was met because someone came in and communicated to headquarters in words he could not express.[2]

So it is with us. When we don't know how to pray, or sometimes even what's wrong, in steps the Holy Spirit. We may not have the words to describe our needs, but our Paracletos knows precisely what we need and He communicates with the Father in words we can't understand. When we don't know how to pray, the Holy Spirit takes over.

Now it's time to put what you've learned into practice. Begin by praying the words of Psalm 139:23-24 to give the Spirit permission to search and know you. Then sit in silence as the Spirit examines your heart and communicates with the Father in words you don't understand. Finally, listen to the Spirit as He encourages, teaches and guides you into all truth.

Father, thank You for sending Your Spirit to communicate my deepest needs to You when I don't know how or what to pray.

Spirit, thank you for interceding on my behalf at the Father's throne. I trust You to ask for exactly what I need.

"Search me, O God, and know my heart; test me and know my anxious thoughts. See if there is any offensive way in me, and lead me in the way everlasting" (Psalm 139:23-24).

Notes
1. William Barclay, *The Apostles' Creed for Everyman* (New York: Harper and Row, 1967), p. 251.
2. Adaptation of a popular story. Original source unknown.

# Group Prayer Requests   Today's Date:_____

| Name | Request | Results |
|------|---------|---------|
|      |         |         |
|      |         |         |
|      |         |         |
|      |         |         |
|      |         |         |
|      |         |         |
|      |         |         |
|      |         |         |
|      |         |         |
|      |         |         |
|      |         |         |
|      |         |         |
|      |         |         |
|      |         |         |
|      |         |         |

# THANKFUL FOR THE PRIVILEGE OF PRAYER

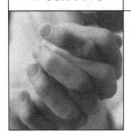

Week Five

MEMORY VERSE

*What other nation is so great as to have
their gods near them the way the Lord our
God is near us whenever we pray to him?*

Deuteronomy 4:7

Before we continue on this journey into a lifestyle of thankfulness, let's review what we have learned thus far. In week one, we learned about God's unfailing love—a love that is good and endures forever. Week two focused on God Almighty, who is our strength in weakness and gives us the ability to sing songs of thankfulness, regardless of our circumstances. During week three, we saw God's compassionate care in action. We can be content and carefree because we are in the loving care of our Good Shepherd. Last week, we saw how God leads and guides us. He does not leave us to face our problems alone, but is always near. By the power of His Holy Spirit, He dwells in our hearts by faith.

Do you see a pattern in this rhythm of thankfulness? Being thankful is not based on outer happenings or material possessions; it is based on the solid foundation of who God is and what He has promised to do for His people. We can always be thankful, even in the worst circumstances, because our Lord has promised to never leave us or forsake us. The God of heaven and Earth, the Mighty One, is near. He leads us and guides us and weaves all things together for our good. We already have sufficient reason to sing God's praise throughout eternity, but there is more!

This awesome God, the creator of heaven and Earth, invites us to converse with Him. Not only does He invite us to pray, He welcomes us into His presence. Have you ever considered what a privilege it is that God invites us to pray? Let's explore this privilege together this week.

# DAY ONE: *Thankful That He Hears Me*

Because prayer is such an important part of our relationship with God, He gives us clear instructions on how we are to pray to Him. Right in the middle of our Bibles there are 150 examples of prayer for us to follow. When we are at a loss for words, we can use these time-honored psalms as our own prayers to God. We will use Psalm 61 as our model for prayer this week. Take time to read the entire Psalm. We will then look at the elements contained in its eight verses.

➤ Verse 1 contains the first element we need to incorporate into our prayers. What did David ask God to do in this verse?

➤ What two common themes do you find in the following verses?

1 Kings 8:30

Nehemiah 1:6

Daniel 9:17

In addition to asking God to hear our prayers, we must humbly ask forgiveness for our sins. Nothing invokes the presence of God faster than the earnest cries of His humble people.

Now it's your turn. Bring to mind a situation that currently burdens you. Compose a prayer in your journal, asking God to help you in your time of need. Begin your prayer by asking God to listen to your words. Acknowledge who God is and who you are in relation to Him, and then clearly state what you need God to do for you. Close by thanking God for graciously hearing your prayer.

 God Almighty, surely Your ear is not too dull to hear the prayers of Your people (see Isaiah 59:1).

"Give ear to my words, O LORD, consider my sighing" (Psalm 5:1).

# DAY TWO: *Thankful I Can Cry Out to Him*

Prayer is not a passive activity. Our God is a passionate God, not a lifeless idol. Our conversations with Him should reflect the life and emotion He has given us.

➤ Turn again to Psalm 61 and read verse 2. Describe David's desires and emotions.

David told God that he was calling out from "the ends of the earth." David was not at home in Jerusalem when he wrote this psalm. He was out of his element and at the end of his rope. His heart was growing weak. He did not feel brave enough to fight. All he wanted was to hide.

➤ According to verse 2, where did David long to be in this moment of utter desperation? Complete David's words to find the answer.

"_____ me to the _____ that is _____ than I."

At the beginning of week three, you wrote down the mental images that the words "Good Shepherd" brought to your mind. Words and phrases that bring up vivid mental pictures are called word bridges; the words form a bridge, or pathway, to our inner thoughts.

➤ What images, emotions and thoughts do the words "rock that is higher than I" produce?

David was not looking for a tall rock to stand on; he was looking for a cave to hide in!

❧ According to Proverbs 30:26, how do coneys (rock badgers), compensate for their powerlessness?

❧ Write Psalm 32:7 in your own words.

❧ Have you ever thought of God as your hiding place—a place into which you can burrow and find safety from storms or enemies? Explain.

❧ How does Psalm 61:2 reinforce what you learned in yesterday's lesson?

❧ End today's lesson by listing the three reasons for thankfulness that you found in Psalm 61:1-2.

   1.

   2.

   3.

Lord God, thank You for allowing me to hide myself in You when I am too weak to fight and too tired to travel on. Thank You for the assurance that I can always find shelter in a rock that is higher than I (see Psalm 61:2).

Thank You, gracious Lord, for words and images that remind me I can make You my hiding place.

## DAY THREE: *Thankful I Can Dwell in His Tent*

The word *selah* appears after many of the psalms. It means "peace" and is an invitation to stop and ponder what we have just read and apply it to our lives.

Read Psalm 61:3-4 and ponder the meaning of those words. The following questions will help stimulate your thoughts.

- David recalled times past when God had been his refuge, "a strong tower against the foe." Recall a specific incident when God was your tower of strength.

- David didn't want to just find refuge from his current dilemma. Where did he long to dwell, and how long did he want to stay there?

- Can you truthfully say that you want to abide in the shadow of God's protective care forever? Or would you rather run to Him in times of trouble and then quickly return to your old ways when the terror of the moment has passed? Explain your answer and why you feel that way.

❧ How does dwelling in God's tents forever apply to consistently following the Nine Commitments of the First Place program?

In the past, we may have gone on rigorous diets when we were trying to look good for an upcoming special event, when we received an ultimatum from someone we cared for, or because of a warning from a health-care professional. Yet when the pressure subsided, our commitment waned.

❧ How is this attitude different from David's desire to make God his refuge forever?

❧ Prayerfully read John 15:1-17 and then compare Jesus' words with what you have learned in today's lesson. How are they connected?

Making a commitment to dwell in God's tent forever is both a one-time choice and an ongoing process. As part of your selah today, spend some time in prayer thanking God that He is a permanent solution, not a temporary fix. Thank Him for inviting you to abide in Him and that He abides in you too. Those who dwell in His shadow are always secure! When you have finished your time of prayer, write one thought in the space below that you can carry with you today.

 O Lord, You alone are my rock and my salvation; You are my fortress, and I will never be shaken (see Psalm 62:2).

Sovereign God, I will trust in You at all times. I will pour out my heart to You, for You are my refuge (see Psalm 62:8).

# DAY FOUR: *Thankful for My Heritage*

On Day 1, we learned the importance of asking God to hear our prayers. Keep this truth in mind as we resume our study of Psalm 61. Read verses 5 through 7 and then answer the questions.

➤ What did David affirm in the first line of verse 5?

➤ Why could David affirm his trust that God had heard his prayer and would answer his petition? Use the words of verse 5 to complete the sentence.

> "For _____ have heard _____ vows, O God; you have given me the _____ of those who _____ your name."

➤ Now write this week's memory verse, Deuteronomy 4:7, in the space below.

➤ After comparing these two verses (Psalm 61:5 and Deuteronomy 4:7), describe the heritage of which David speaks in Psalm 61:5.

Our heritage as God's chosen people allows us to come to God, our heavenly Father, as dearly loved children who are always welcome in His presence.

➣ According to Hebrews 4:16, how are we encouraged to approach God? What will we receive when we do so?

➣ David declares that this heritage belongs to those who fear God's name (see Psalm 61:5). How can we fear God's name and still come boldly into His presence? Aren't fear and boldness contradictory? Explain.

Whenever we find seemingly contradictory statements in Scripture, we must look for a deeper meaning to the words that, at first glance, appear to disagree.

➣ First John 4:16-18 tells us that fear has to do with punishment. What is the perfect love that casts out fear?

➣ Read Isaiah 53:4-6. Why don't those who are in Christ Jesus need to fear God's wrath any longer?

To check your answer, read John 3:36. What assurance is found in this verse?

Using the foundational truths found in John 5:24 and Romans 8:1, express your thanks to God. Come boldly into His presence, because Jesus Christ died to give you the privilege of coming before God in prayer. God's name is no longer a source of fear for those who are in Christ Jesus!

Gracious God, thank You for loving me and sending Jesus to take on my sins so that I can have the privilege of crying out to You in prayer.

Precious Lamb of God, You were without spot or blemish, yet You willingly bore all of my sins and died in my place so that I can be in a right relationship with my heavenly Father. Your perfect love takes away my fear of God's punishment.

## DAY FIVE: *Thankful I Can Sing His Praise*

David ended Psalm 61 with a bold declaration. Write Psalm 61:8 in the space below exactly as it appears in your Bible.

Because of what God had done for David, David promised to do two very specific things as a sign of his gratitude. Look back over the words you wrote above and circle those two specific actions.

First, let's look at these two actions individually. Later, we will combine the two and apply them to our lives.

⋙ How is singing praise to God's name similar to living a life characterized by thankfulness? Are they one and the same? Explain.

⋙ Summarize David's words in 2 Samuel 24:24.

What might it cost you to offer God a sacrifice of thanksgiving? What would you have to give up in order to live a lifestyle of thankfulness? Perhaps negative music keeps you in defeat and despair, or a toxic relationship drains your energy and vitality. Maybe He requires you to give up a disordered relationship with food. Be sure to give this question very careful thought, because you cannot truthfully answer the next question until you have done so.

≫ Is this a cost you are willing to pay? Why or why not?

≫ Returning to the second part of David's statement in Psalm 61:8, how is fulfilling your vows day after day part of the First Place program?

≫ Can you see a connection between giving an offering of thanksgiving to God and fulfilling your vows every day? Explain.

≫ How is being faithful to the First Place program commitments both a sacrifice and a reason for singing praises to God?

≫ How will a lifestyle of thankfulness help you to fulfill your commitment to First Place day by day?

Now go back and reflect on all you have learned this week. Summarize the lessons in your mind. Offer God a sacrifice of thanksgiving by listing all the reasons this lesson has given you to sing praises to God, your permanent dwelling place and refuge from the storms of life. In your words of praise, also express thankfulness for the privilege of prayer.

"O God, you are my God; earnestly I seek you. I will praise you as long as I live, and in your name I will lift up my hands" (Psalm 63:1,4).

You are awesome, O God. You give power and strength to Your people. Praise be to You (see Psalm 68:35).

## DAY SIX: *Reflections*

The book of Psalms was the foundation of Jesus' prayer life, and it can be yours too. Even as our dying Savior hung on the cross in mortal agony, Jesus prayed psalms (compare Psalm 22:1 with Matthew 27:46, and Psalm 31:5 with Luke 23:46). When all other language failed, psalms were the default language Jesus relied on to express His thoughts. We saw this same default language in week two of our study; Mary and Hannah (Day 2) and Paul and Silas (Day 3) relied on the words of Scripture prayers to see them through tough times.

If you are new to the book of Psalms, it may seem a bit confusing. At first glance, the psalms appear to be a jumble of praise, thanksgiving, lament, confession and assurance. In our Western society, we are used to having material presented in a much more orderly fashion—or at least categorized for us under subheadings! We are used to a linear thought process that goes from point *A* to point *B* to point *C*, after which we expect to see a neat and orderly conclusion. One of the valuable lessons we learn from the psalms is that our lives are not always neat and orderly. Life doesn't always proceed from point *A* to point *B* to point *C* in a predictable fashion. Rather than a straight path, our lives often resemble a switchback trail up the side of a steep mountain. If our prayer lives are to be consistent, our prayers must accommodate the full range of emotions and circumstances that define our lives.

Psalm 66, a psalm of thanksgiving, is closely related to many of the lessons we have learned this week. Read this psalm and then make a list of all the things you find to be thankful for in the words of this Scripture prayer. Pay particular attention to verses 13 and 14. Think of the vows you made to God when you were in distress—vows you quickly forgot when the storm clouds went away.

End today's reflections by making Psalm 66:20 your own prayer. Write those awesome words on an index card and read them often throughout the day. Maybe you would even like to commit them to memory.

How awesome are Your deeds, O God! So great is Your power. I will sing to the glory of Your name and offer You glory and praise (see Psalm 66:2-3).

"Let the righteous rejoice in the LORD and take refuge in him; let all the upright in heart praise him!" (Psalm 64:10).

"But as for me, it is good to be near God. I have made the Sovereign LORD my refuge; I will tell of all your deeds" (Psalm 73:28).

## DAY SEVEN: *Reflections*

During our Day 2 study, we learned about the concept of word bridges.

≫ In your own words, describe what word bridges are and the type of bridge they form.

Throughout Scripture, God uses word bridges—simple words or phrases that act as pathways to thoughts, emotions and images. These word bridges can teach us powerful truths about God and how He cares for His people. Listed below are some word bridges that God uses to teach us about Himself. Beside each word bridge, write the thoughts, emotions and images it produces in your mind. Since we used the word bridge "rock that is higher than I" in Day 2, you can use that as your starting point.

| Word Bridge | Thoughts, Emotions and Images Evoked |
|---|---|
| "The rock that is higher than I" (Psalm 61:2) | |
| "My shield" (Psalm 18:2) | |
| "[My] help" (Psalm 33:20) | |
| "My fortress" (Psalm 59:16) | |

There is an important principle we must learn when allowing Scripture word bridges to bring up thoughts, emotions and pictures. We must first understand the context of a word bridge before we allow it to make pathways into our minds. Consider the following example of two very different uses of the same word.

≫ How is the word bridge "stronghold" used differently in Psalm 27:1 and in 2 Corinthians 10:4?

A good rule is to read a few verses before and after the sentence in which you see the word bridge so that you will clearly understand the image the writer intended to portray through his words. Whenever you see a word bridge in Scripture, remember the little word "selah." Stop and let the thoughts, feelings and images the writer intended to evoke fill your heart and mind. Then thank God for giving you His Word in a language you can understand.

I love You, Lord. You are my strength, my rock, my fortress and my deliverer (see Psalm 18:1-2).

O Lord, You preserve the faithful. I will be strong and take heart because I put my hope in You (see Psalm 31:23-24).

I sing praise to You, O my strength, my fortress and my loving God (see Psalm 59:17).

# GROUP PRAYER REQUESTS   TODAY'S DATE:_____

| NAME | REQUEST | RESULTS |
|---|---|---|
| | | |
| | | |
| | | |
| | | |
| | | |
| | | |
| | | |
| | | |
| | | |
| | | |
| | | |
| | | |
| | | |
| | | |
| | | |

# THANKFUL FOR DARK DAYS

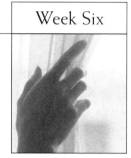

MEMORY VERSE
*You, O Lord, keep my lamp burning; my*
*God turns my darkness into light.*
Psalm 18:28

Last week we looked at the command to offer God a sacrifice of thanks-giving. Equating sacrifice (which we view as painful) with thankfulness (which we picture as pleasant) is a difficult concept. The key to under-standing this principle is to choose to thank God for dark days. When the dark clouds descend like a thick blanket, we must not forget that God is in the business of developing character; and character, like film, develops best in the dark! As wonderful as the sunny mountaintop experiences are, without dark days, we will never develop into mature men and women who reflect the image of Christ.

Before we begin this week's lesson, write Proverbs 3:5, Jeremiah 29:11 and this week's memory verse on a sheet of paper. When you have fin-ished writing the verses, read them aloud, and then begin Day 1. Reread the verses aloud before the start of each lesson this week. (You may want to fold the paper to fit inside this book as a reminder.)

## DAY ONE: *Thankful for Precious Promises*

Dark days have many sources. Scripture tells us that sometimes, dark days are the result of testing so that our faith can be purified and refined. Other times, they are a form of temptation the enemy sends our way, or a result of others' actions—intentional or unintentional. There are as many rea-sons for dark days as there are dark days; but they all have one thing in common, regardless of their origin: All dark days feel awful!

During this Bible study, we have learned about word bridges.

≫ What feelings, emotions and thoughts does the phrase "dark days" evoke?

Feelings spring from our fallible thought processes; however, facts are based on the infallible Word of God. The book of James describes people who base their faith on their feelings rather than on the truth of God's Word.

≫ Turn to James 1:2-8 and complete the following sentence:

"Consider it pure _____, my brothers [and sisters], whenever you face _____ of _____ _____" (v. 2).

≫ According to James, why do we face trials of various kinds (vv. 3-4)?

≫ Is James's statement based on fact or feeling? How do you know?

≫ James tells us that testing produces _____ (v. 3). What is the end result of this quality (v. 4)?

≫ What can you ask God for so that you will not be left in the confusion and doubt these various kinds of trials produce (v. 5)?

Can you expect a favorable response to your request? Why or why not?

➤ In verses 6 through 8, James paints us a word picture that describes a person who bases his faith on feelings. Describe the picture these verses paint in your mind.

➤ The apostle Peter gives us the antidote for this instability that you just described. Turn to 2 Peter 1:3-4. What is Peter's prescription for times of trial?

How does Peter describe God's promises? What do God's promises allow us to do?

Which of God's great and precious promises do you need to cling to today so that you can be faithful to the Nine Commitments of First Place?

Thank You, gracious Lord, for Your great and precious promises that serve as my anchor during troubling times (see 2 Peter 1:4).

Lord, You have promised to give wisdom to all who ask. Today I ask You for wisdom so that I can safely navigate troubled waters (see James 1:5).

# DAY TWO: *Thankful God Is in Control*

Did you remember your reading assignment? If not, reread the verses that you wrote on sheet of paper on Day 1 (Proverbs 3:5; Jeremiah 29:11; Psalm 18:28).

Perhaps the most vivid example of testing in the entire Bible is found in the book of Job. Read Job 1—2 now to get an overall picture of Job's situation.

➤ What does God say about Job in 1:8?

Have you ever had people tell you that your troubles and trials were the result of something you were doing wrong? Now, certainly unconfessed sin can have dark consequences, but Job 1:8 makes it clear that even when we are right with God, we may still be tested. We should not assume that dark days in our lives, or in the lives of others, are a result of sin.

➤ Yesterday, we learned that God uses trials to test our faith. According to James 1:13, does God also tempt us?

God perfects our faith through trials, but Satan attempts to destroy our faith through temptation.

➤ Turn back to Job 1—2. What was Satan trying to prove about Job's faith in Job 1:9-11 and 2:4-5?

To understand the connection between testing and temptation, consider the new-car road-test commercials you see on television. The maker of the automobile being tested uses this trial to show just how good their automobile really is. Conversely, the competition uses the road-test results to prove the same car is flawed.

How does this comparison relate to our testing by God and temptation by Satan?

What would happen if you treated temptation as an opportunity to pass the test and prove to Satan that the power in you is greater than all his deceptive tricks?

God allowed Job to be tested so that Job would be proven faithful; Satan tempted Job to prove that Job's profession of faith in God was false.

How might this analogy relate to your participation in First Place?

According to Job 1:12 and 2:6, what limits did God give Satan?

God set a limit on what Satan could do to Job, and He will set a limit on your testing too. You will not be tempted beyond your ability to withstand the trial (see 1 Corinthians 10:13). Remember, God wants to refine you, not crush you. Isaiah 42:3 is a precious promise that you can cling to in troubled times. Perhaps you would like to write it on the paper with the other three verses you are reading aloud each day.

 Lord God Almighty, thank You for allowing me to maintain my integrity and prove my love for You during times of trial (see Job 2:3).

You will not break an already damaged reed, and You will not snuff out a smoldering wick. Thank You for the assurance that You limit my trials and temptations so that I can bear them (see Isaiah 42:3; 1 Corinthians 10:13).

# DAY THREE: *Thankful He Hovers Over Me*

In week five, Day 7, we looked at words God uses in Scripture to portray various aspects of His nature. One image that was not on our list can be found in the following Scriptures:

➣ How is God portrayed in the following verses?

Ruth 2:12

Psalm 91:3-4

Matthew 23:37

When the storm clouds appear and we run around like frightened little chickens, God takes us under His wings and shelters us from the storm. Left to our own devices, we would run straight into the fowler's snare! Pause for a moment and thank God, the mother hen, that He allows you to find shelter under His almighty wings!

We are all familiar with the image of the dove, which is often used to portray the Holy Spirit. But there is another image of the Holy Spirit in Scripture that you might not be as familiar with.

➣ Turn to Genesis 1:2. What was the Spirit of God doing?

According to verse 3, what happened next?

➣ Have you ever pictured the Spirit of God hovering over your dark days, partnering with God the Father to bring clarity to your confusion and light to your darkness? Explain.

How does this image reinforce the lesson we learned in week four, Day 7?

≫ Write this week's memory verse below. You have been reading it out loud every morning this week, so perhaps you can write it from memory!

How does Psalm 18:28 connect with what you just read in Genesis 1:2-3 and what you studied yesterday in Isaiah 42:3?

≫ God alone turns your darkness into light! Write a prayer of thankfulness to the Holy Spirit for hovering over you during dark days and for bringing light to the empty darkness that is about to bring forth new life.

 Almighty God, thank You for saving me from the fowler's snare and for sheltering me under Your wings (see Psalm 91:3-4).

Spirit of the living Lord, You hovered over the formless earth. Hover over my confusion and darkness and bring forth light, clarity and new life (see Genesis 1:2-3).

# DAY FOUR: *Thankful for Discipline*

Sometimes our dark days are a result of God's discipline. What we mistake for God's anger is really a sign of His love! Most of us are familiar with the wonderful picture of the cloud of witnesses that surrounds us as described in Hebrews 12:1, but when we get to the part about sin and opposition and discipline, we quickly turn to another page. Today, discipline yourself to read the entire passage of Hebrews 12:1-13.

➤ Verses 5 and 6 are quoted from Proverbs 3:11-12. Paraphrase these verses in your own words.

Why should we not make light of the Lord's discipline or lose heart when He rebukes us? What does His discipline prove (see Hebrews 12:6; Proverbs 3:12)?

➤ In week five, Day 4, we learned about our heritage as children of God. How is God's discipline also part of that heritage?

➤ Hebrews 12:10 repeats a truth we learned earlier this week. Compare this verse to what you learned in Day 1. How are they complementary?

➤ Does the writer of Hebrews pretend that discipline is pleasant while it is happening (v. 11)?

In Day 1, we talked about feelings versus facts. Compare the feelings we experience in testing with the truth about God's discipline as found in verses 10 and 11.

*How do the facts about God's discipline apply practically to keeping the Nine Commitments of First Place?

The apostle Paul gave us another insight into God's discipline. Read 1 Corinthians 11:31-32. In these verses, "judged" means being found in need of discipline, akin to the judgment that takes place when a test we have taken reveals that we still have areas of weakness that need to be corrected.

*Describe the correlation between self-discipline and God's discipline based on these verses.

*Now, apply that truth to the First Place program. If you don't want God to find you lacking and in need of His discipline, what must you do?

*What can you do today to make self-discipline part of the godly training you are receiving through the First Place program?

⇛ How can God's discipline be a source of profound gratitude and part of the lifestyle of thankfulness we are developing through this Bible study?

Loving Father, although Your discipline doesn't always feel good, I know that it is a sign of Your love for me and proof that I am part of Your family.

Lord Jesus, thank You for being my example, so that I will not grow weary and lose heart during times of trial (see Hebrews 12:3).

## DAY FIVE: *Thankful for Rainbows*

After 40 days and 40 nights of heavy rain, the downpour finally stopped. Although the earth had been destroyed by the great flood, Noah and his family were kept safe and dry inside the ark that Noah had constructed in obedience to God's command. Yet even though the rains had finally stopped, Noah and his family were not on dry land yet.

⇛ According to Genesis 7:24, how long after the 40 days of rain was the earth flooded? (This will require some math!)

⇛ Use the words of Genesis 8:3 to complete the sentence below.

"The water receded _____ from the earth."

What can we learn from that word about the process of recovering from a personal disaster or time of intense testing?

Recovery is a process, not an instantaneous event. God could have dried up the water immediately, but He chose to teach Noah more about His faithfulness through a steady process of events that eventually led Noah to dry land.

≫ As a pledge of His promise to never flood the earth again, God put a sign in the sky. According to Genesis 9:8-17, what was the sign, and what did it signify?

God put a beautiful sign in the sky as a seal of His covenant promise to Noah. Genesis 9:9-10,12 tells us that Noah was not the only one included in the covenant that God sealed with a rainbow.

≫ List the other people and things that are covered by God's promise.

No matter what trial you are presently facing, after the rain there will be a steady process of recovery, followed by a beautiful rainbow. God's mercies are new every morning. Take heart. You will not be consumed.

 Faithful Father, if it were not for Your great love, I would be consumed. Thank You for Your faithfulness and merciful love (see Lamentations 3:22-23).

Today, Lord, I am thankful for rainbows, sunrises and sunsets, which all remind me that You are a God of new beginnings who always brings new life out of darkness, no matter how bleak the night.

# DAY SIX: *Reflections*

At the beginning of the week, you were asked to write three Scripture verses on a piece of paper and to read these verses aloud before you began each day's lesson. Perhaps you have been wondering why you were asked to read them aloud. Although we usually read Scripture silently, God's Word is intended to be read, heard and taken to heart (see Revelation 1:3). Even in private settings, we benefit from reading a text aloud because it allows us to take the words in through two senses— sight and hearing—rather than one. When we read silently, we tend to read quickly, often skimming and skipping over words that bring depth and meaning to the passage. When we read verses out loud, we often hear ourselves speaking just the words of wisdom we need to hear in that moment. We become our own encouragers when we tell ourselves the story of God's perfect love.

Psalm 46 is a powerful reminder of God's present help in time of trouble. Turn to this psalm and read it aloud in a way that portrays the passion and drama embodied in these words. Every time you see the word "selah," stop and think about what you just read. When you come to verse 10, do exactly what the psalm instructs you to do: Be still and know that God is who He says He is.

End your reflections with a prayer of gratitude to the Lord Almighty, who is always with you. The God of Jacob is your fortress! Let your thankfulness overflow.

Merciful Father, my comfort in suffering is this: Your promises renew my life (see Psalm 119:50).

O Lord, Your Word gives light to my feet when I travel dark paths (see Psalm 119:105).

Sovereign Lord, recounting Your words gives me light and understanding (see Psalm 119:130).

# DAY SEVEN: *Reflections*

Since the horrific events of 9/11, the entire world has been in a heightened state of alert. Disaster preparedness and homeland security have taken on new dimensions and higher priorities. Emergency relief agencies now need to be prepared for more than natural disasters like earthquakes, hurricanes, tsunamis, floods and fires. We are all more conscious of the need to keep a storehouse of emergency supplies to tide us over in the event of a catastrophe. But there is another type of disaster preparedness that the public doesn't talk much about: a storehouse of supplies for the spiritual disasters of life. Two of the First Place commitments prepare us for such emergency situations and build up a storehouse of spiritual rations to see us through times of inner chaos and disaster.

Our first spiritual supply is the Word of God, which we have safely tucked into our hearts for such times. We have a ready reserve of verses from which we can draw any time a need arises. We need only ask the Holy Spirit to bring to our mind those great and precious promises we have stored away. The Spirit knows exactly which ones we need at any particular time. He goes swiftly to our cupboard and brings just what we need to see us through any emergency.

Our second spiritual provision is prayer. Praise God that we do not need to come to Him in times of need as strangers. Through consistent daily prayer, we have developed an intimate relationship with the true and living God. We can come to Him boldly and ask for assistance in our time of need because we are confident that He hears and answers our prayers. We don't know when disaster will strike, but we can always be prepared. When we are diligent to stock our spiritual storehouses with God's emergency rations, we will never be found lacking.

Spend time recalling the disaster preparedness verses you have hidden away in your spiritual survival kit. If you find your cupboard is getting bare, recommit yourself to the memory verse commitment. God's Word is the oil that keeps your light burning and allows you to weather the darkness of even the blackest night.

O Lord, though the waters roar and foam, and the mountains fall into the sea, You are my refuge and my strength, an ever-present help in times of trouble (see Psalm 46:1-2).

You, O Lord, are the everlasting light. Shine in my life throughout eternity (see Isaiah 60:19).

Lord Jesus, You are the light of the world. You keep my lamp burning; You turn my darkness into light (see John 8:12; Psalm 18:28).

# GROUP PRAYER REQUESTS   TODAY'S DATE:_____

| NAME | REQUEST | RESULTS |
|------|---------|---------|
|  |  |  |
|  |  |  |
|  |  |  |
|  |  |  |
|  |  |  |
|  |  |  |
|  |  |  |
|  |  |  |
|  |  |  |
|  |  |  |
|  |  |  |
|  |  |  |
|  |  |  |
|  |  |  |
|  |  |  |

# THANKFUL FOR GOD'S WORD

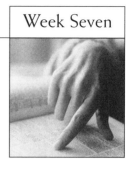

Week Seven

MEMORY VERSE
*I rejoice in following your statutes*
*as one rejoices in great riches.*
Psalm 119:14

The apostle Peter gives us yet another jewel to add to our treasure chest of thankfulness. Second Peter 3:2 says, "I want you to recall the words spoken in the past by the holy prophets and the command given by our Lord and Savior through your apostles." If you have faithfully kept your thankfulness journal for the past six weeks, you have probably made several entries thanking God for the riches found in His Word. However, few of us think to give thanks for the faithful men and women throughout the ages who have made it possible for us to receive this incredible gift.

⟫ Using 2 Peter 3:2 as a guide, make a list of those who have made it possible for you to receive the Word of God. Include those specifically listed in the text and any others you can think of.

   Did you remember to include the printers, publishers and booksellers who make the Word available to you in written form, and the instructors who taught you how to read it?

## DAY ONE: *Thankful for Proclaimers*

In Ephesians 4:11-13, the apostle Paul lists four specific types of servants that the living Lord has sent to His Church.

⟫ List the four types of spiritual gifts listed in verse 11.

1.

2.

3.

4.

⇒ Why are these special gifts given to members of the Church? What is their ultimate purpose (v. 12)?

God has sent these spirit-filled messengers to His Church so that we can be prepared for service. Through their faithful proclamation of God's Word, the Body of Christ is equipped to serve, united in purpose, growing in knowledge of the Son of God, and becoming mature Christian men and women. Quite a gift indeed!

⇒ These powerful proclaimers were called to spread God's Word in a very dynamic way. How does Paul describe his calling in 1 Thessalonians 2:4?

Paul was _____ by God and _____ with the Gospel.

Recall the person who introduced you to First Place. Thank God for sending this special messenger into your life. As an expression of your gratitude, tell your First Place story to someone who is still struggling with out-of-control eating. When you have reached your target weight, be sure to send your testimony via e-mail to the First Place national office so that your story can be part of the message that proclaims God's truth to those in need of a healthy lifestyle.

Thank You, Father, for sending apostles, prophets, evangelists and pastor-teachers to proclaim Your Word and to help me grow in Christian maturity so that I can serve You with wholehearted devotion.

Gracious God, thank You for sending powerful pro-claimers to spread the gospel. Today I am especially thankful for the ministry of First Place.

## DAY TWO: *Thankful for Encouragers*

Yesterday's lesson focused on powerful proclaimers of the Word of God. Today we will look at another word ministry that God uses to spread the gospel. Turn back to 2 Peter 3 and refer to verses 1 and 2 to answer the following questions:

➤ How did Peter greet his readers?

➤ What two reasons prompted him to write this personal letter to his friends?

➤ What would we call someone who stimulates others to wholesome thinking?

Peter did not claim to be giving new information. He was not impart-ing some new wisdom or teaching. His purpose in writing his friends was to motivate and encourage them to recall what had already been spoken.

➣ Look up the word "wholesome" in a dictionary. Based on this definition, describe the kind of thinking Peter was trying to stimulate in his readers' minds.

How is wholesome thinking part of the First Place program?

➣ Encouragement is one of the Nine Commitments of First Place. What can you learn from Peter's words that will help you stimulate your First Place friends to wholesome thinking?

Our encouragement should be warm, sincere and based on the Word of God—not on our own thoughts and opinions.

➣ Write this week's memory verse below.

Recall the people you listed in this week's introduction who made it possible for you to receive God's Word. How have those people become a reason for you to rejoice in the vast riches found in God's Word?

Close today's lesson by thinking of someone who has stimulated you to wholesome thinking by encouraging you to remember God's truth. Make a note of that person in your thankfulness journal and then write that person a letter expressing your thankfulness for his or her warm, sincere encouragement. Encouragers need encouragement too!

My Lord and my God, I want to live a healthy, balanced life that honors You and inspires others to become part of a First Place group. Thank You for sending First Place friends to encourage me to think wholesome thoughts.

Merciful Father, forgive me for the times I try to impose my thoughts and opinions on others rather than directing them to the spiritual riches that are only found in Your Word.

## DAY THREE: *Thankful for Humble Instructors*

Proclaimers and encouragers are not the only people God sends to equip His disciples for ministry. Today we will read about two very special people who made a valuable contribution to the Early Church by using their gifts to strengthen a fellow worker.

➤ Read Acts 18:18-26. Not including Paul, we are introduced to three new characters in the exciting saga of the Early Church. What were their names?

Apollos was a powerful proclaimer. He had many attributes that were needed by the Early Church. Verses 24 through 26 tell us about some of these special abilities. If you have a Bible dictionary, look up "Alexandria" to get a better understanding of the cultural heritage of this learned man.

➤ Yet for all his strengths (and they were many!), Apollos had one serious limitation. What was his weakness (v. 25)?

Although Apollos was speaking boldly, he was speaking without knowing all the facts. He had incomplete information. However, God provided two humble instructors to help Apollos.

➣ What did Priscilla and Aquila do for Apollos (v. 26)?

What godly characteristics did Priscilla and Aquila possess that prompted them to invite Apollos into their home and privately teach him the truth?

Apollos went on to become a key figure in the Church. Some Bible scholars even believe that Apollos was the author of the book of Hebrews.

➣ What might have happened to Apollos's ministry had Priscilla and Aquila handled this delicate situation differently?

Priscilla and Aquila were tentmakers, yet Luke tells us that they knew "the way of God" and were willing to explain it to Apollos "more adequately" (v. 26).

➣ What characteristics did Apollos possess that allowed him to willingly listen to these two humble tentmakers, who probably didn't have his educational background or dynamic speaking ability?

If you had Priscilla and Aquila with you right now, what truth about God's Word would you ask them to explain to you?

Ask God to send a humble instructor to explain the Word to you more adequately and to give you the information you need to serve Him effectively.

>>> Read Colossians 3:12. Paul describes five qualities with which all Christians should clothe themselves. What were these qualities and how were they evident in Priscilla, Aquila and Apollos?

Think of an instructor who took you aside and explained the way of God to you more adequately. Maybe it was a Sunday School teacher, a youth pastor or a First Place friend. Write a letter to that person, sharing what he or she did for you and how his or her instruction allowed you to serve God more effectively. After you write the letter, add that person's name to your thankfulness journal.

Father, thank You for the humble instructors You have placed in my life to lead me into Your truth. May I be ready to do the same for anyone You place in my path.

Sovereign Lord, clothe me in compassion, kindness, humility, gentleness and patience, for I am Your dearly loved child (see Colossians 3:12).

## DAY FOUR: *Thankful for Leaders*

As we begin today's lesson, reflect on what you have learned so far this week. Write a short paragraph describing how God's Word has come to you through the special people the Holy Spirit has faithfully brought into your life.

❧ How are these people a sign of God's faithfulness—and a reason for thankfulness?

❧ Hebrews 13:7 tells us about another type of person who brings God's Word to us in a unique way. What group of people is described in this verse?

What two methods did these people use to communicate the gospel to their followers?

❧ After reading the brief description given to us in Hebrews 13:7, do you think these leaders had learned the joy of keeping God's statutes? Explain.

Read Luke 11:37-44 to see how these loving leaders were different from the Pharisees Jesus criticized.

❧ How were the Pharisees that Jesus rebuked similar to the uncaring shepherds we learned about in week three?

❧ How are the leaders we learn about in Hebrews 13:7 a reflection of the Good Shepherd?

In Hebrews 13:7, we are not only exhorted to listen to what these loving leaders have to say. We are also told to:

"_____ the outcome of their way of life
and _____ their faith."

≫ Recall this week's memory verse. If a leader were to equate keeping God's commands with possessing great riches, how would this attitude persuade you to imitate his or her faith?

≫ Now read 1 Corinthians 4:14-17 and Philippians 4:9. Summarize what Paul said in these verses in two words.

≫ Does the way you live your life preach the gospel in word and in deed? Could you encourage others to "imitate" you because of how diligently you keep the Nine Commitments of First Place? Why or why not?

As you have done at the conclusion of the previous lessons this week, recall a person who has modeled the message of God's love to you. Thank God for giving you such a godly example to imitate, and then write a thank-you note to the loving leader who taught you by example what it is like to be a messenger of the gospel.

Thank You, dear Lord, for sending men and women to model the message of Your love and to preach the gospel in word and deed.

Gracious God, I pray for all those who lead by loving example. Keep them in Your tender care.

# DAY FIVE: *Thankful for Storytellers*

When we begin listing the people who bring us God's Word, it is easy to forget one very special type of messenger: the storyteller. Through their talent and imagination, these gifted people make the gospel come alive for us in new and exciting ways.

➤ Write a synopsis of your favorite Bible story, along with the reference, in the space below. Following the story, tell why this event has had special meaning in your life and what lessons you have gleaned from reading this account.

Deuteronomy 6:4-9 gives specific instructions to God's people. Turn to this passage and read the words aloud.

➤ What specific commands did God give His people in this passage? Begin with the command to hear.

➤ Deuteronomy 6:6 tells us the commandments are to be on our _____. What First Place commitment helps you to faithfully keep this command?

➤ When were the Israelites to talk about what God had commanded (v. 7)?

➤ What is one of the most effective ways to impress God's Word on the hearts of the children in your life? (It is the subject of today's lesson!)

➤ Recall a specific Bible story that someone took the time to impress on your heart when you were a child. What one thing about this story impressed you most? (If you were not exposed to Bible stories when you were young, recall one of the stories you learned as a spiritual child.)

Is this the same story you listed at the beginning of this lesson?

Think of a storyteller who brought God's Word to you in a special and unique way. Perhaps this person was a Sunday School teacher, a member of a Christian theater group, or someone who shared their personal testimony in a way that touched your heart and gave you new insight into God's Word. Add that person to your thankfulness journal. Now, as you have done before this week, write that person a thank-you note.

➤ How can storytelling be part of keeping God's statutes so that you have reason to rejoice?

➤ How can storytelling be incorporated into your new lifestyle of thankfulness?

Gracious God, today I thank You for storytellers. Their ministry has touched my heart and brought Your message to me in special and unique ways.

Help me to tell the story of Jesus and His love as I sit at home and as I walk along the road. Help me to treasure Your Word in my heart so that I can give an answer whenever I am asked about my faith and trust in You (see Deuteronomy 6:7).

## DAY SIX: *Reflections*

Yesterday we were reminded that storytellers bring God's Word to us in easy-to-understand ways. Jesus was a master storyteller; throughout the Gospels, He told simple, earthly stories to illustrate powerful Kingdom principles. Do you recall what these earthly stories with heavenly meanings are called? (Matthew 13:10 will help to refresh your memory.)

➤ Read Matthew 13:11-17 to learn why Jesus spoke in parables. What do you find in this passage that you need to incorporate into your lifestyle of thankfulness?

The fact that you have been given eyes to see and ears to hear the truth of God's Word is a gift more precious than great riches!

One of the simple parables that Jesus told involved a man and a hidden treasure. Take note of the italicized words:

> The kingdom of heaven is like treasure hidden in a field. When a man found it, he hid it again, and then *in his joy* went and sold all he had and bought that field (Matthew 13:44, emphasis added).

➤ How is the parable that Jesus told similar to this week's memory verse?

If you were the man in Jesus' parable, would you be willing to sell everything you owned to obtain the riches found in keeping God's statutes? Would doing so give you great joy? Reflect on this question throughout the day.

You are my Lord and my God. "I would rather be a doorkeeper in [Your house] than dwell in the tents of the wicked" (Psalm 84:10).

O Lord, "I delight in your decrees; I will not neglect your word" (Psalm 119:16).

Whoever trusts in material wealth will fall, but those who are in a right relationship with You, O God, will thrive like green leaves (see Proverbs 11:28).

# DAY SEVEN: *Reflections*

One of the emotions that we must deal with when we begin to bring our out-of-control eating under the lordship of Jesus Christ is deprivation. Once we commit ourselves to the First Place program, the battle begins. Suddenly, the things we can't have take on a life of their own! Cookies call from the cupboard; ice cream screams from the freezer; the candy jumps right out of the dish. The "forbidden fruit" becomes our preoccupation. That's when the evil one seizes the opportunity to convince us that God is withholding something good that we deserve. From the beginning, Satan has used feelings of deprivation as part of his arsenal of deception when tempting God's children to go outside the boundaries that God has established for our welfare.

The wise words of Proverbs 15:32 tell us the truth: "[The one] who ignores discipline despises himself." God's Word tells us that self-discipline is not deprivation. As a matter of fact, Scripture tells us that self-discipline is the hallmark of self-care. The *lack* of discipline is true deprivation. We despise ourselves when we ignore God's limits and boundaries that protect our health and well-being. We deprive ourselves of God's abundant blessings when we insist on doing life our way rather than surrendering our will to His. God gives grace to the humble, and humility has no feelings of deprivation because it has no sense of entitlement (see Proverbs 3:34).

Humility says that God knows what is best for us and that He will not withhold anything good from those whom He loves. Humility delights in the Lord, trusting that as we do things His way, He will give us the desires of our hearts.

In our backward society, rejoicing and obedience seem opposite. Even some of those who keep God's statutes often try to portray themselves as self-made martyrs. They live lives characterized by self-deprivation and struggle; but what does our memory verse tell us about those who keep God's commands?

They are _____ and they _____!

Being spiritually rich and filled with joy are treasures that no amount of money can buy. Use the following questions as fodder for your journal writing today. Talk to Jesus about your inner thoughts and listen as He shares His heart with you.

- How are spiritual riches an integral part of a lifestyle of thankfulness?
- How is self-discipline part of your storehouse of spiritual treasure that money cannot buy?
- Do you find joy and delight in being obedient to God's Word? If not, why?

O Lord, Your commands are more precious to me than pure gold; they are sweeter than honey straight from the comb. By Your Word I am warned of danger, and I will be rewarded for obeying You (see Psalm 19:10-11).

Father, keeping your statutes is my joy and my delight (see Psalm 119:14).

O Lord, I am blessed when I keep Your statutes and seek You with all my heart (see Psalm 119:2).

# GROUP PRAYER REQUESTS  TODAY'S DATE:_____

| NAME | REQUEST | RESULTS |
|---|---|---|
|  |  |  |
|  |  |  |
|  |  |  |
|  |  |  |
|  |  |  |
|  |  |  |
|  |  |  |
|  |  |  |
|  |  |  |
|  |  |  |
|  |  |  |
|  |  |  |
|  |  |  |
|  |  |  |
|  |  |  |

# THANKFUL FOR GOD'S GRACE

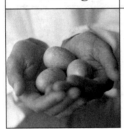

## MEMORY VERSE

*He who did not spare His own Son, but gave him up for us all—how will he not also, along with him, graciously give us all things?*
Romans 8:32

The apostle John ended his eyewitness account of the good news of Jesus Christ with these telling words: "Jesus did many other things as well. If every one of them were written down, I suppose that even the whole world would not have room for the books that would be written" (John 21:25). Similarly, to thoroughly explain grace, the subject of this week's study, would require more pages than this world could contain, and it would take all of eternity just to complete this week's lesson!

While the subject of grace is a river so deep and wide and high that it is inexhaustible, it can also be summed up in three little words.

➤ Write Titus 3:5 below. Once you have written it, underline the first three words. Now write those three words in large, bold print, substituting the word "me" for "us."

Those three words contain the amazing truth about grace!

As you complete this week's lessons, you will soon be able to paraphrase John's words to read, "If I were to list all the reasons I have to be thankful for God's grace, there would not be enough room in the whole world to contain the thankfulness journals that I would fill!"

## DAY ONE: *Thankful He Lifted Me from the Pit*

> Amazing grace! How sweet the sound!
> That saved a wretch like me!
> I once was lost, but now am found;
> Was blind, but now I see.[1]

John Newton penned the words of the beloved hymn "Amazing Grace" more than 200 years ago, but his words still ring true in the hearts of those who have been saved by God's amazing grace. The words are as precious to believers today as they were to John Newton. However, because language has changed over the past 200 years, there is one word you may not fully understand. This word is the starting point to understanding God's amazing grace.

➣ Look up the word "wretch" in your dictionary and write its meaning below. You may paraphrase the definition in your own words.

➣ How does Revelation 3:17 expand on the definition you just described?

What was the discrepancy between how the Laodiceans saw themselves and how God saw them?

This is the beginning of grace: When we are given eyes to see our pitiful condition, we begin to see things from God's point of view and can then appreciate what He has done for us.

⟫ How did David describe his pitiful condition in Psalm 40:2?

⟫ During weeks three and four, we learned about word bridges. What thoughts, feelings and images do you associate with "slimy pit"?

Although we can use phrases like "slimy pit" to describe our wretched condition without blinking an eye, it is much more difficult to be down-and-dirty honest about how things really were before God saved us. When we give our public testimony, we may speak in general terms; but in our private time before God, we must tell ourselves the whole truth. Until we get to the nitty-gritty of our former life, we will never realize the full extent of God's amazing grace.

Since this is a First Place Bible study, spend some time remembering just how wretched your condition was before God saved you from your powerful addiction to food. When your thoughts materialize, write them down in your prayer journal.

Gracious and merciful God, I am amazed at the depths of Your love. While I was a sinner, You died for me (see Romans 5:8)!

Lord God Almighty, there is just no way my finite mind can grasp the deep riches of Your amazing grace. You redeemed me from the slimy pit. Jesus saved me!

## DAY TWO: *Thankful for God's Solution*

Once we begin to grasp our pathetic condition—the "how it was" part of our story—we need to quickly move on to "what happened." To wallow in the slimy pit is not the purpose of our confession. Confession means to agree with God. Once we have acknowledged that we are not rich, wealthy or self-sufficient but "wretched, pitiful, poor, blind and naked," we are ready to move on to the next step (Revelation 3:17). Praise God! Before He gives us eyes to see the problem, He has already provided the solution to our distress.

➤ In the introduction to this week's lesson, you were asked to summarize God's grace in three words. Write those words again now.

➤ Read Paul's declaration about God's solution in Romans 7:24-25. Make these words your own by rewriting them in the space below in your own words.

➤ Turn back to Titus 3:3-8. Use Paul's words to briefly describe:

How it was (v. 3)

What happened (vv. 4-6)

How life is now (vv. 7-8)

Now it's time to apply this passage to your own life. The following summary will help you give an answer to others who ask you what you are doing to lose weight. Later, you can use this outline to write your First Place testimony.

➤ Using the same format, write a brief description of your First Place story.

How it was


What happened


How life is now


➤ Use Titus 3:4 to complete the following phrase:


"_____ when the _____
and _____ of God our _____ appeared."


➤ What did we learn in week two, Day 5, about the transitional word "but"?




Just as David turned his lament into thankfulness by remembering God's faithful love, you can do the same in your salvation story. Go back to your outline above. In the margin to the left of your outline, write Titus 3:4, and then personalize the text by changing "our" to "my."

➤ Who is Paul referring to when he writes about the kindness and love of God your Savior? Write His name in bold letters!




➤ Reword Titus 3:4 into a statement of thankfulness. Write it here and in your thankfulness journal.

Lord Jesus Christ, You are the goodness and kindness of God, who appeared to save me from my sins. Your grace is amazing and my heart is grateful (see Titus 3:4).

Thanks be to You, almighty God! Through Jesus Christ my Lord, I have been rescued from a life of self-destruction (see Romans 7:25).

## DAY THREE: *Thankful That Jesus Saved Me*

We began Day 1 with a hymn about God's grace. Sing those wonderful words again. If you have a hymnbook, you might want to sing more than just the first verse.

Philippians 2:6-11 was a hymn of the Early Church. It was probably sung as part of worship, much like we sing "Amazing Grace" today. Go to that passage now and read it slowly, letting the words fill your heart and mind.

➤ Which verse in this passage resonates most in your heart? Write it in the space below.


What about this verse makes it especially meaningful for you?


The very fact that Jesus was willing to make Himself nothing, to take the nature of a servant and come to Earth in human flesh, is beyond our finite minds. Now add to that staggering truth the fact that Jesus humbled Himself and became obedient to death—even death on a cross. If the story stopped right there, we could all exclaim, "Amazing grace!" and live a lifestyle of thankfulness just basking in those words. However, the wonder does not stop there.

➤ At the beginning of this week's study, we looked at Paul's words in Titus 3:5, "He saved us." Remember what you were asked to do with those words? Write them again below.

How does personalizing Paul's words make grace all the more amazing?

Pause for a moment and ponder the amazing fact that had you been the only sinner on the face of the earth, Christ still would have gone to the cross for you. Augustine put it this way: "God loves each of us as if there were only one of us."[2] That amazing fact alone is ample reason to give thanks!

Turn to Ephesians 2:8-10. These words are a wonderful example of grace in action. We will study this passage more carefully tomorrow; however, before we look at these words in detail, answer the following questions and ponder them throughout the day.

➤ How is grace defined (v. 8)?

Why can you never boast (v. 9)?

Why did God save you (v. 10)?

➤ Today's lesson has given us lots of food for thought. How might digesting God's amazing grace be part of the solution to your out-of-control eating? You can write your answer here or in your prayer journal.

My Lord and my God, how can I ever begin to thank You for what You have done for me? When I was lost in my sin, You saved me!

Gracious God, sometimes I worry about my future. Help me to always remember that You sacrificed Your Son for me. When I ponder that fact, how can I doubt Your gracious provision for all my other needs (see Romans 8:32)?

## DAY FOUR: *Thankful I Can Respond*

Toward the end of yesterday's lesson, you were asked to read Ephesians 2:8-10. Now that you have pondered those words overnight, go back and reread them.

Many Christians confuse justification and sanctification, and because they aren't clear about what these terms mean, they don't understand what grace is all about.

➤ Justification is a one-time event. According to Paul's words in Ephesians 2:8-9, is there anything you can do to earn salvation? Why?

If you could earn God's grace, it would no longer be a gift; rather, it would be a wage.

➤ Turn to Romans 6:23. As a sinner, what are your just wages?

➤ According to this week's memory verse, Romans 8:32, who paid the price so that you could receive justification as a free gift?

In essence, what are you doing when you try to earn your salvation?

If we could earn our salvation, we would have reason to boast. We would not be totally dependent on the grace of God.

➤ Last week we learned about parables. Turn to Luke 12:16-21. In one sentence, summarize Jesus' message about depending on our own accomplishments.

Unlike justification, which is a one-time event, sanctification is a process of becoming more like Christ, which begins the millisecond we confess Him as our Lord and Savior and continues until we go home to spend eternity with God. Paul tells us in Philippians 2:12 that we are to

"_____ _____ [our] _____ with fear and trembling."

Does this seem contradictory to grace? Not if you understand what Paul was saying. Paul was not saying that we work *for* our salvation; he was saying that we work *out* our salvation.

➤ One of the First Place commitments is exercise. What is the purpose of a physical workout?

Through exercise you develop, strengthen and tone your muscles. In weeks six and seven, we learned that God's goal is to make us mature, complete and lacking in nothing. However, we must cooperate with the process. We must exercise our spiritual muscles, nourish our minds and hearts with His Word, and grow in grace and knowledge so that we will develop perseverance, endurance and strength. While our efforts do not contribute one iota to our *justification*, they are very important to our *sanctification*.

➤ How is First Place part of your sanctification process? Are you working out your salvation by keeping the Nine Commitments of First Place?

➤ Remember, you are God's handiwork. He created you for a purpose. How is self-care part of the response grace demands?

 Forgive me, Father, for those times I rely on the work of my own hands instead of kneeling in humble gratitude before the One who saved me!

Help me, gracious Lord, to work out my body and my spirit so I can be whole and complete, lacking nothing. Grace demands a response. Today I say yes to You!

## Day Five: *Thankful for Grace upon Grace*

As you have learned this week, grace is a free gift from God. You cannot work for it; you cannot earn it. You must accept it as God's gift to you, because the moment you try to earn it, you negate your faith in Jesus Christ. Once you have received God's grace, you have all the grace you need. There are no degrees of grace with regard to justification. Justification is an all-or-nothing proposition.

Another Scripture passage that sometimes brings confusion until we understand it properly is 2 Corinthians 12:9. We already looked at this verse briefly during week two, but read it again now and then complete the sentence below.

"My _____ is sufficient for you, for my _____
is made perfect in _____."

We know that Paul was not saying he needed to be saved a second time. He was not implying that his thorn in the flesh indicated that he had fallen out of God's grace. Paul was a champion of the sufficiency of Christ's atonement. Once Jesus stretched out His arms on the cross and cried, "It is finished," there was absolutely nothing else required.

Paul was reminding himself and the Corinthians that grace, like many other mysteries of the Christian life, is both a one-time gift and an ongoing process. We are saved by God's grace, and as we go through the sanctification process, God gives us ongoing grace to do everything He has purposed for us to do.

➤ Write this week's memory verse, Romans 8:32.

What words in this verse show us that grace is a one-time event?

What words reveal to us that grace is an ongoing process?

God didn't save us and then leave us to flounder on our own. Recall our week four, Day 4, lesson. What was God's promise, as found in Deuteronomy 31:6 and Joshua 1:5?

"He will never _____ me nor _____ me."

✎ Are you currently struggling with a problem that seems too heavy to bear? What does this week's memory verse promise you?

Remember, God had the solution before you were even aware of the problem!

✎ What can you do today to allow God's grace to be sufficient for you and His strength to be made perfect in your weakness as He completes the work He began in your life? Be sure to include the Nine Commitments in your answer.

 You, O Lord, are able to keep me from falling and to present me before Your glorious presence without fault and with great joy. My only God and Savior, to You be glory, majesty, power and authority, through Jesus Christ my Lord, before all ages, now and forevermore! Amen (see Jude 24-25).

## DAY SIX: *Reflections*

Exactly as the name implies, word bridges serve as a bridge between what is written on the page and the pictures with which our mind is already familiar. Mental pictures truly are worth a thousand words! This is why skilled communicators use word bridges rather than endless verbiage to give life to their message.

✎ In the space below, list all the thoughts, pictures and emotions that the word "riches" brings to your mind.

Perhaps you have seen the following acrostic used to explain grace:

God's
Riches
At
Christ's
Expense

≫ How do the words in this acrostic compare with your descriptions of riches from the previous question?

Did you picture riches in strictly physical terms? When we limit riches to the physical realm, Scripture appears to contradict itself, because not all Christians are rich in material possessions. As a matter of fact, Jesus and His apostles warned against the danger of depending on physical wealth.

≫ Read 1 Timothy 6:6-19. Summarize Paul's words to Timothy in a sentence or two.

≫ How are God's riches, purchased for you at Christ's expense, part of a lifestyle of thankfulness?

 Gracious God, earthly riches do not endure forever, but Your love will last throughout eternity. Therefore, I will put my hope and trust in You.

O Lord, give me neither poverty nor riches, but give me only my daily bread. I know that You will not withhold any good thing from me because You gave up Your own Son on my behalf (see Proverbs 30:8; Romans 8:32).

Merciful Father, I know that godliness combined with contentment is great gain. Help me to be content in Your love (see 1 Timothy 6:6).

## DAY 7: *Reflections*

Write out the following two verses. If you have completed *Giving Christ First Place*, the first book in the First Place Bible study series, perhaps you can write both verses from memory.

Matthew 6:33

Romans 8:32

These verses contain one common phrase. Underline it in both verses.

"All things" is an all-inclusive phrase. In the spaces below, list some of the "all things" you have received in each category as a result of giving Christ first place through your participation in the First Place program.

| Physical | Emotional |
|---|---|
| Mental | Spiritual |

⤜ First Place is a program of balance. Are your "all things" lists balanced among all four areas? If not, what can you do to enjoy God's riches equally in all areas of your life?

The last verse in "Amazing Grace" has been all but forgotten. The words are printed below. You began this week singing the first stanza of this beautiful expression of grace; end the week by singing these wonderful words.

> The earth shall soon dissolve like snow,
> the sun forbear to shine;
> But God, Who called me here below,
> shall be forever mine.[3]

Add that marvelous fact to your thankfulness journal!

 Lord Jesus Christ, You deserve first place in my life. Help me to honor You through my faithfulness to the First Place program.

Gracious God, I am Your handiwork. Today I will care for my body because You care for me (see Ephesians 2:10).

My Lord and my God, Your love is beyond my comprehension. When I had done nothing to deserve Your love, You redeemed my life from the pit! Thank You for Your amazing grace.

Notes
1. John Newton, "Amazing Grace," *Then Sings My Soul* (Nashville, TN: Thomas Nelson, 2003), p. 78.
2. Saint Augustine, quoted in http://www.quotedb.com/quotes/217 (accessed April 28, 2005).
3. John Newton, "Amazing Grace," p. 79.

# GROUP PRAYER REQUESTS   TODAY'S DATE:_____

| NAME | REQUEST | RESULTS |
|------|---------|---------|
|      |         |         |
|      |         |         |
|      |         |         |
|      |         |         |
|      |         |         |
|      |         |         |
|      |         |         |
|      |         |         |
|      |         |         |
|      |         |         |
|      |         |         |
|      |         |         |
|      |         |         |
|      |         |         |
|      |         |         |

# THANKFUL FOR ETERNAL HOPE

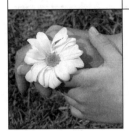

## MEMORY VERSE

*Therefore, since we are receiving a kingdom that cannot be shaken, let us be thankful, and so worship God acceptably with reverence and awe.*
Hebrews 12:28

Have you ever read a book so suspenseful that, when all seemed hopeless and lost, you turned to the back of the book to see how it ended? Then, knowing the ultimate outcome, you were able to continue reading, confident that whatever happened on the pages between now and the end, things would turn out okay. Knowing the ending made the uncertainty of the moment bearable.

God, in His grace, has done the same thing for us. He assures His children that no matter how traumatic the present might be, a happy ending lies on the horizon: We will be with the Lord forever (see 1 Thessalonians 4:17). No matter how hopeless the present moment may seem, Jesus Christ has overcome the enemy, and because we believe in Him, we will share in His victory.

➤ Let the words of John 16:33 permeate your being. Read the verse, and then complete the following statements:

Jesus wants us to have _____. In this world we will have _____, but we can take _____ because He has _____ the world!

# DAY ONE: *Thankful for My Future Home*

Before Jesus went home to be with His Father in heaven, He assured His disciples that He was not leaving them alone. Recall what you learned in week four, Days 4 and 5 about the One who God sent to take Jesus' place.

➤ Who came to take His place?

How was it to the disciples' advantage to have Him present?

Jesus sent His Spirit to reside in the disciples' hearts. He would never again be limited by a physical body. In the Spirit, Jesus could be with all His disciples at the same time.

➤ How does this amazing fact affect the way you live your life, especially with regard to First Place?

You need never fear that God is too busy doing other things to be available to you. He is intimately involved in every aspect of your life. He doesn't play favorites, so there is absolutely no need for competition or rivalry.

➤ Read Psalm 139:7-12. What do these verses confirm?

Jesus also informed His disciples what He would be doing for them once He was back in heaven with His Father. Read John 14:1-4 to answer the following questions:

≫ What was Jesus' first command to His disciples (v. 1)?

What made it possible for them to keep this command?

≫ What had Jesus gone to His Father's house to do (v. 2)?

≫ Once He had done this, what would He do (v. 3)?

It has often been said that the goal of Christianity is not to get us into heaven, but to get heaven into *us*. Jesus is not only preparing a place for you through the process we discussed last week—sanctification—He is preparing you for that place! The master carpenter is carving out a niche for you and whittling you down so that you will fit into that special place.

≫ How is God using First Place to fit heaven into you and to make you fit for heaven? (Don't limit your answer to physical size!)

Thank Jesus for preparing a place for you—and for preparing you for that place. Both are part of a lifestyle of thankfulness.

Thank You, Jesus, for using Your Spirit and Your Word to prepare me for the wonderful place that You are preparing for me!

Sovereign Lord, thank You for the assurance that I will
be with You forever. Yes, there will be trouble in this world,
but I will take courage, because You have overcome the world.
How grateful I am that You have allowed me to read the end
of the book to give me the assurance that I have a future full
of hope (see John 16:33).

## WEEK TWO: *Thankful for Vision*

Toward the end of his life, the apostle John was exiled to the island of
Patmos. Turn to Revelation 1:9 and read why John was sent away to this
desolate place.

❧ Why was John exiled to the island of Patmos?

While on that lonely island, John still held fast to the truth and wor-
shiped the Lord, even though he was no longer part of the congregation
at Ephesus that had been his place of ministry for many years. The letters
we now call 1, 2 and 3 John tell of this faithful shepherd's love and concern for his flock.

❧ Imagine for a moment that you are exiled to a remote island, separated from your church family and friends, because of your faithfulness
to the Word of God. Describe the emotions and thoughts you might
feel in that situation.

During John's time on the island of Patmos, some of his friends were
allowed to visit him and take the letters John had written back to the
mainland. These letters were then read to the congregations to strengthen

and encourage them in John's absence. One day a very special messenger came to visit John.

➤ According to Revelation 1:1-2, who came to John and why?

➤ Having received this special vision from God, what did John do (v. 19)?

➤ Look at Revelation 1:3 and Revelation 22:7,10. Why do you think it is so important to God that we read, hear, take to heart and obey what He revealed to John in this vision?

Reading the book of Revelation is a lot like reading the last page of a suspenseful book so that you can read the remaining pages in the light of the happy ending that awaits you. Thank God for eternal hope!

➤ How is the First Place program part of reading, hearing, taking to heart and obeying the Word of God?

➤ What blessings have you received by being faithful to the Scripture reading and Bible study commitments of First Place? Make your answer a statement of heartfelt gratitude.

Thank You, Lord, for preparing me for the things that are to come so that I can be assured of the outcome. I will hold fast to the knowledge that I will be with You forever.

Gracious God, thank You that the apostle John was faithful to Your command and recorded what he saw. Now I can be prepared for the hour of Your return, which is ever imminent. Help me also to be faithful in the things You ask me to do while I eagerly await Your triumphant return.

## DAY THREE: *Thankful for Messengers*

Yesterday, you learned about the apostle John's circumstances when the angel came to him on the island of Patmos.

➤ Read Revelation 1:4-5. Who sent the angelic messenger to John?

This is a message from the Trinity! Look closely to see how the triune God is described.

➤ How is God the Father described (v. 4)?

The sevenfold Spirit before the throne (v. 4) is the Holy Spirit in all His fullness, not seven separate spirits.

➤ How is Jesus, the Son, described (v. 5)?

At the beginning of a book, an author usually dedicates the work to someone special as a way of thanking that person for the valuable contribution he or she made to the life of the writer.

※ The book of Revelation also contains a dedication. Using Revelation 1:5-6 as a guide, fill in the blanks to discover the recipient of this special dedication.

"To him who _____ us and has _____ us from our _____ by his _____, and has made us to be a _____ and _____ to _____ his _____ and _____—to him be _____ and _____ for ever and ever! Amen."

※ To whom is the book of Revelation dedicated?

Stop for a moment and let that incredible truth sink in. This is a book written by the Trinity and dedicated to Jesus Christ. In His love and compassion, God is preparing us for the events that will take place at the end of this age. This should be enough to make all believers overflow with thankfulness.

※ Think back to yesterday's lesson about the circumstances in which John wrote this message. What does this tell you about how God can use our trials to His glory and to ultimately benefit His faithful children?

"Be at rest once more, O my soul, for the Lord has been good to you" (Psalm 116:7).

Father, today I worship You with reverence and awe. You are the One who is, who was, and who is to come (see Revelation 1:4).

# DAY FOUR: *Thankful for Correction*

It has been said that the role of prophecy is to comfort the afflicted and afflict the comfortable. Nowhere do we see this principle more clearly illustrated than in the book of Revelation.

The message John received while on Patmos was directed to seven churches located in Ephesus, Smyrna, Pergamum, Thyatira, Sardis, Philadelphia and Laodicea. Although these were seven literal churches in Asia Minor, Bible scholars agree that the message delivered to these churches is for the entire Church. The message to us is as important as it was to the actual seven churches named. Though we will not have time to study each of the messages God sent to the seven churches, you might want to read each of them to see how His warnings apply to you. You will find these messages in Revelation 2—3. If you are interested in learning more about the conditions addressed in these letters, you can use a Bible dictionary to learn about the ancient cities themselves.

The purpose of the letters to the seven churches was not condemnation. In our modern language, we would call these messages wake-up calls.

➣ Summarize the messages given in Revelation 2:7,11,17,26-29; 3:5-6,12-13,21-22.

Our gracious Lord was giving the churches—and gives the modern Church—a chance to repent and turn back to Him before it is too late.

➣ How does Revelation 2—3 correspond to what we learned about God's discipline in Hebrews 12:5-13?

➣ How is the First Place program part of God's wake-up call to you?

Remember, this is not about condemnation. This is a correction sent by a God who loves you and wants only good things for you. His loving correction signifies that you are a valuable member of His family.

Add to your thankfulness journal the fact that God loves you enough to warn and correct you.

Father, I am thankful that You love me enough to discipline and correct me. Give me ears to hear and eyes to see the wake-up call that You are giving to me through the First Place program.

Gracious Lord, help me not to lose heart when You correct me. Rather, help me to see Your discipline as a sign of Your mercy, compassion and love.

## DAY FIVE: *Thankful for Redemption*

While we receive God's correction, we can find hope in knowing that He does not hold our sins against us. Hebrews 12:29 tells us that our God is a consuming fire, but in His mercy and love He sends that fire to purify—not to destroy—those who have been called according to His purpose.

➤ Lamentations 3:22-25 is a promise we can cling to when our world is spinning and we feel that we cannot endure. Write this promise below. You might want to add this reassurance to your storehouse of memory verses.

➤ In week four, Day 1, we learned that Jesus is both the Good Shepherd and the Lamb of God. What does 1 Peter 1:18-19 tell us about the blood of the Lamb?

➣ Look up the word "redeem" in a dictionary and paraphrase this definition in a few words.

➣ Now read Hebrews 9:28. How is this truth related to our memory verse and to our eternal hope?

Jesus Christ is our atonement. He will return a second time, not as a sacrifice for our sin, but to fulfill His promise of eternal salvation to those who are waiting for His return. Praise God that you are among the redeemed! You were enslaved to sin and destined to death, but Jesus paid the price for your freedom. He became your substitute so that you could be free. He lived a sinless life and then took all of your sins so that you can be right with God. Maybe you want to stop right now and sing the first and last stanzas of "Amazing Grace" again!

Recall the lessons we learned in week eight about God's grace. Can you understand now why it is so important to be painstakingly honest about "how it was"? Until you come to terms with the life from which Jesus redeemed you, you can never be fully thankful for the depth of His love. There is no such thing as "cheap grace." Jesus Christ gave His life so that you can spend eternity with God.

➣ Read 1 Corinthians 6:19-20. According to verse 20, how should we respond to the grace we have been given?

How does the First Place program help you to show your gratitude toward God for His grace?

How might knowing that you have been redeemed by the blood of the Lamb be part of a lifestyle of thanksgiving?

I love You, O Lord, for You heard my voice; You heard my cry for mercy (see Psalm 116:1).

Lord Jesus Christ, I was once far from God, but now I have been brought close to Him through the sacrifice of Your precious blood. You purchased my peace with God at a very high price (see Ephesians 2:13-14).

# DAY SIX: REFLECTIONS

One of the foundational principles of logic is the proposition "If P, then Q," or (P → Q). In such a proposition, either both facts are true or both facts are false; there cannot be a false P and a true Q, or vice versa. In logical progression, for Q to be true, P must have occurred. Throughout Scripture God makes "If . . . , then . . . " propositions that we often erroneously confuse with God's promises. We try to claim the "then" without first fulfilling our part of the bargain, and we become disappointed when the promise that we are trying to claim does not take place. In order to claim the benefit, we must first do the work. Propositions only become promises when we do our part.

The following chart lists several verses that contain "If . . . , then . . . " propositions. Look up the verses and complete the chart. In some verses, both the "if" and the "then" are clearly stated; in other verses, one or both are implied. Not every proposition carries a positive outcome—if we do the "if" in these situations, the "then" won't be very pleasant!

| Scripture | If | Then |
|---|---|---|
| Deuteronomy 11:22-23 | | |
| Joshua 24:20 | | |
| 2 Chronicles 7:14 | | |
| Proverbs 2:1-9 | | |
| Matthew 6:33 | *You seek first the kingdom of God and His righteousness* | *All these things will be given to you as well.* |
| Luke 9:23 | | |
| John 6:51 | | |
| John 8:36 | | |
| 1 Corinthians 3:17 | | |
| 1 John 1:7 | | |

First Place is also an "If . . . , then . . . " proposition. *If* we put God first in all things and follow the Nine Commitments of First Place consistently, *then* we will reap the rewards of a balanced, healthy life. You cannot expect the benefits of First Place if you have not done the work!

≫ Which of the Nine Commitments of First Place are you keeping on a consistent basis?

Which of the commitments are you failing to keep, while still expecting to reap the benefits of this program?

Now create your own "If . . . , then . . . " chart based on the tenets of First Place and write some positive and some negative outcome statements. For example, "If I eat according to the Live-it Plan, then I will achieve my goal weight" or "If I do not exercise, then my body will not be strong and sleek." Try to pick an "If . . . , then . . . " statement for each commitment.

| If | Then |
|---|---|
| | |
| | |
| | |
| | |
| | |
| | |
| | |

Take time today to ask yourself a logical question: Am I expecting God to do His part when I have not been willing to do mine? Faith includes doing our part, faithfully following the Nine Commitments of First Place, confident that God will keep His end of the bargain.

 O Lord, I will humble myself and pray and turn from my sinful ways so that You can bring health and healing to my life (see 2 Chronicles 7:14).

Jesus Christ, You are the Bread of Life. If I eat of this bread, I will live forever (see John 6:51).

Thank You, gracious Father, for Your promises. Because I walk in the light, I can be confident that the blood of Jesus, Your Son, purifies me from all sin (see 1 John 1:7).

## DAY 7: *Reflections*

If you have completed Wellness Worksheet Two, you have probably realized that there are as many different ways to express thankfulness as there are individual Christians. Yesterday's reflection was designed for those of us who express and process our thoughts in a logical mathematical thankfulness style. Other reflections throughout this study have been created for those who process thankfulness in different ways. Today's reflection is designed for those who thank God best through body movement.

The wonderful thankfulness expressed in Psalm 100 is printed at the end of this section. Read these words over several times so that you become familiar with them. Once you have the flow of the words, try repeating this psalm in different body positions: kneeling, sitting and standing with your face to the heavens and arms extended skyward. (If you have physical limitations that prohibit any of these postures, adapt them to fit your body's abilities.) Make note of how your body posture affects the way the words sound as they go through your body. What emotions does each position evoke?

≫ Kneeling

≫ Sitting

≫ Standing with arms outstretched

Read the psalm aloud once more. This time, pause after each sentence and pose your body in positions that express the meaning. Hold the pose for 20 to 30 seconds before moving on to the next sentence. Now do this exercise again, this time moving from one posture to the next in a fluid motion.

Finally, walk around the room in a march-like cadence, repeating the psalm in time to your steps. As you march, imagine you are part of the triumphant procession marching behind Christ, the King.

**Psalm 100**
Shout for joy to the LORD, all the earth.
  Worship the LORD with gladness;
  come before him with joyful songs.
Know that the LORD is God.
  It is he who made us, and we are his;
  we are his people, the sheep of his pasture.
Enter his gates with thanksgiving
  and his courts with praise;
  give thanks to him and praise his name.
For the LORD is good and his love endures forever;
  his faithfulness continues through all generations.

 God Almighty, I will enter Your gates with a thankful heart and Your courts with praise (see Psalm 100:4).

Thank You, Father, for allowing me to praise You however my heart feels led. Teach me to listen to Your Spirit's prodding.

You, O LORD, are good, and Your love endures forever! I praise You because Your faithfulness continues throughout all generations (see Psalm 100:5).

# GROUP PRAYER REQUESTS    TODAY'S DATE:_____

| NAME | REQUEST | RESULTS |
|------|---------|---------|
|      |         |         |
|      |         |         |
|      |         |         |
|      |         |         |
|      |         |         |
|      |         |         |
|      |         |         |
|      |         |         |
|      |         |         |
|      |         |         |
|      |         |         |
|      |         |         |
|      |         |         |
|      |         |         |
|      |         |         |

# A LIFESTYLE OF THANKFULNESS

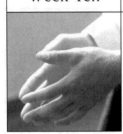

MEMORY VERSE
*Always giving thanks to God the Father for every-*
*thing, in the name of our Lord Jesus Christ.*
Ephesians 5:20

Thankfulness is a conscious choice that you must make based on who God is and what He has done for you. You do not have to rely on the shifting tide of emotions and circumstances for your thankfulness. God has given you everything you need to be faithful to His command to "give thanks in all circumstances, for this is God's will for you in Christ Jesus" (1 Thessalonians 5:18).

If you have faithfully kept your thankfulness journal over the past nine weeks, you have already begun to reap some of the rewards that come from giving God thanks for all the little things you previously overlooked. In the weeks ahead, you will continue to reap abundant blessings. Perhaps you have also read Carole Lewis's book *A Thankful Heart*, which applies many of the thankfulness principles you have learned in this study. Carole relates powerful stories from her own life and from the lives of other First Place members that serve as practical examples of thankfulness lived out on a daily basis.

## DAY ONE: *Thankful I Can Choose*

Thankfulness is not only a lifestyle, but it is also a choice; the very fact that we can choose is a profound reason for thankfulness. When God created Adam and Eve, He gave them free will. They had the freedom to choose whether or not they would obey God. However, when sin entered the world, their freedom turned into slavery—slavery to sin. A right relationship with God was no longer a choice they could make on their own.

Adam and Eve hid from God because they suddenly felt naked and ashamed (see Genesis 3:8-10). Sin shattered paradise and all of creation fell under a curse.

Do you remember the "If . . . , then . . . " exercise we did on Day 6 last week? Turn to Genesis 2:16-17. After reading the passage, turn God's words into an "If . . . , then . . . " proposition.

| If | Then |
| --- | --- |
|  |  |

The logic of "If P, then Q" goes back to the beginning of creation. From the time Adam and Eve disregarded God's clear command, humanity has reaped the consequences of their folly. We are only able to have right relationships with God because Jesus Christ was willing to come to Earth, live a sinless life and die in our stead.

➤ What does 1 Corinthians 15:21-22 reveal about the differences between Adam and Jesus Christ?

➤ Second Timothy 2:25-26 reveals a truth about our freedom to choose. To whose will are we captive until the Son sets us free?

➤ In Romans 8:5-8, Paul gives us a very clear picture of the difference between those ruled by the Spirit and those caught in Satan's web. Compare Paul's descriptions of these two types of people below.

Ruled by the Spirit

Ruled by sin

➳ Read Romans 6:16-18. What do you learn from these verses? Can the natural man or woman (those under the curse of the Fall) please God? Explain.

Praise God that Jesus Christ came to set us free from our bondage to sin and death! We are no longer held in Satan's snare, captive to his will. Jesus died to restore our freedom to choose life.

➳ What did Jesus say about the freedom He gives, as recorded in John 8:36?

➳ Based on what you have studied today, why are you able to make wise choices?

Only those who have been redeemed from a life of sin and death are able to live a lifestyle of thankfulness. Thank God that His Son has set you free so that you can choose thankfulness, which pleases God.

 Thank You, gracious Father, for sending Jesus to restore my freedom of choice. Today I choose You!

O Lord God, how dependent I am on You. Even my ability to choose is a result of Your goodness and grace. You have set me free, and I am free indeed (see John 8:36).

## DAY TWO: *Thankful for Process*

Just as we grow in physical stature and strength from childhood to adulthood, our Christian formation—becoming more and more like Christ—is also a process of growth. Our Christian maturity, just like physical growth, can be measured.

Turn to 1 John 2:12-14. John divides the Christian growth process into three categories: dear children, young adults and mature fathers and mothers of the faith. Use the chart below to list the characteristics of each maturity level.

| Children | Young Adults | Fathers and Mothers |
|---|---|---|
|  |  |  |

Can you see the progression? Basic belief in Jesus leads to strength to overcome evil, which leads to deep intimacy with God.

Basic faith ⟶ Overcome evil ⟶ Deep intimacy

⇒ On a scale of 1-10, with 1 being basic belief in Jesus and 10 being deep intimacy with God, where would you rate your level of Christian maturity?

| 1 | 2 | 3 | 4 | 5 | 6 | 7 | 8 | 9 | 10 |
|---|---|---|---|---|---|---|---|---|---|

Basic belief                     Intimacy with God

Second Peter 5-8 lists a formula for growth and maturity. Peter told his readers, "If you possess these qualities in increasing measure, they will keep you from being ineffective and unproductive in your knowledge of our Lord Jesus Christ" (v. 8).

⇒ Turn to 2 Peter 1:5-8 and complete the following sequence laid out by the Apostle as the pathway to Christian maturity:

Faith + _____ + _____ +

_____-_____ + _____ +

_____ + _____ _____ +

Love = Christian Maturity


In what measure does Peter say that we are to possess these qualities (v. 8)?




Once we have gone through the progression, we cycle back through it, growing in grace and knowledge each time we make the loop. In a world characterized by downward spirals, Peter's formula presents us with a way to grow up in our faith.

➤ Read on to 2 Peter 1:9. How does Peter describe those who do not possess these qualities?




Now, let's apply this same upward spiral model to the Nine Commitments of First Place.


Attendance + E_____ + P_____

+ Bible _____ + Scripture _____

_____ + _____ study + _____-____ plan

+ C_____ R_____ + E_____

= First Place Success


Like Peter's equation, the First Place commitments also need to be practiced in increasing measure!

Now apply the progress theory to a lifestyle of thankfulness. Drawing from the main thought that you have gleaned from each of the nine lessons on thankfulness thus far, complete the following equation:

God's _____ Love + _____
Strength + _____ Compassionate Care +
God's _____ + P_____
+ _____ Days + G_____ W_____ + God's
+ _____ Hope = A Lifestyle of Thankfulness

A lifestyle of thankfulness is also attained in increasing measure. Little by little, step by step, we learn to trust God and, in the process, overflow with thankfulness.

Review all three equations. In each of the equations, draw circles around the areas in which you are weak.

➣ What can you do to add to each of these categories in increasing measure?

Christian maturity

First Place success

A lifestyle of thankfulness

Take one step toward each goal today!

Thank You, Father, for allowing me to know what is pleasing to You. Today I pray for the wisdom and the power to take the next step so that I can grow closer to You and live a life of thankfulness that brings glory and honor to Your holy name.

O Lord, You do not leave me to my own devices. You have given me Your Word so that I can chart my course and measure my progress. Thank You for being a God of great mystery, yet a God of predictable results.

# DAY THREE: *Thankful for Contentment*

Yesterday, we focused on growth and progress. However, we can never become so focused on our destination that we lose sight of the present joys. In the Christian life, there exists a tension between the promise of tomorrow and the enjoyment of today. We strive for excellence and add to our progress in increasing measure; yet we find joy and contentment in today.

"Contentment" is not a popular word, mainly because it is often confused with complacency.

≫ Look up "contentment" and "complacency" in a dictionary and write each definition below.

Contentment—

Complacency—

In your own words, explain the difference between the two.

Both words mean "satisfied." But look more closely at "complacency." Where does the satisfaction come from? "Contentment" means "being satisfied with what one has," while "complacency" means "being satisfied with oneself." The rich fool described in Luke 12:16-21 was complacent. He was smug in his own accomplishments and did not need God. Read his story again. Can you see his complacent smugness?

≫ Turn to the following verses to discover the sources of the Christian's contentment. Write your discoveries in the spaces provided.

Philippians 4:11-12

1 Timothy 6:6-7

Hebrews 13:5

Contentment is being satisfied with God and His gracious material provisions and providential care; it is not a smug self-satisfaction that feels it no longer needs God. As we strive to grow in our Christian faith, we have the present assurance that God will give us everything we need to accomplish His purposes for us.

Many of us who are not content were raised by parents whom we could never fully please. Instead of reprogramming our thoughts, we transfer the not-good-enough attitude of our childhood to other people, places and situations in adulthood. If you come from such a background, take a long, hard look at contentment. Perhaps God is using this study as your wake-up call. No matter how often you verbally affirm God's greatness or how many praise songs you sing, you will never realize the joys of living a lifestyle of thankfulness until you make contentment part of that lifestyle.

→ How is contentment part of the First Place program?

→ What can you do today to be more content with your life, with God and with the provisions He has given you?

Gracious and loving Lord, I trust in Your provision for my every need. Though my flesh and my heart may fail, You will be the strength of my heart and my portion forever (see Psalm 73:26).

Father, never allow me to get so complacent that I feel I have no need for You. Remind me that I am only self-sufficient because of Christ's sufficiency.

# DAY FOUR: *Thankful for New Beginnings*

First Place is a program of new beginnings. No matter what happened yesterday, today is the first day of the rest of your life!

≫ Turn to Philippians 3:12-14 and prayerfully read Paul's words. Summarize this passage below.

Now turn to Acts 9:1-14, in which Paul describes a part of his past that he needed to leave behind in order to run the Christian race unhindered.

≫ What was Paul doing before Christ met him on the Damascus road (vv. 1-2)?

Was Paul's reputation common knowledge among believers (v. 13)?

≫ What was Ananias's main concern about going to see Paul (v. 14)?

We can certainly understand why Paul would need to leave that part of his past behind in order for him to move forward. However, there was another part of Paul's past that he considered garbage when compared with knowing Christ.

≫ According to Philippians 3:4-11, what other aspect of Paul's past did he have to leave behind?

What was the most important thing in the world to Paul (vv. 8-10)?

When we come to the First Place program, we must learn to be like Paul and treat each day based on its own merit. We cannot allow ourselves to dwell on the painful parts of our past, nor can we gloat over past accomplishments. Each day, we must keep the Nine Commitments as if we were beginning the first day of the rest of our lives. We must let go of the hurts that wound and the pride that puffs up if we are going to press on toward the prize.

➼ Go back to Philippians 3:12 and complete the following statement:

> Paul was striving to take _____ of that for which Christ Jesus had taken _____ of him!

In that wonderful play on words, Paul relays a valuable spiritual truth. Stop and think about his statement for a moment.

➼ Why has Christ taken hold of you? Are you striving to take hold of the very thing He freed you to achieve?

➼ Are you willing to let go of the past so that you can take hold of your future in Christ Jesus and achieve all that He has in store for you? What can you do today to begin the process?

Father, thank You for new beginnings! Help me to leave the past behind so I can grasp the wonderful things You have in store for me.

Were it not for Your great love, O LORD, I would be consumed. Because of Your mercy and compassion, each morning brings new mercies. Great is Your faithfulness (see Lamentations 3:22-23).

## DAY FIVE: *Thankful for First Place*

Until this week, we have focused on who God is and what He has done for us. As stated in the introduction to week one, the secret to giving thanks in all things—even those dark days we don't understand—is found in Psalm 77:11-12. David cried out in his anguish and pain, "I will remember the deeds of the LORD; yes, I will remember your miracles of long ago. I will meditate on all your works and consider all your mighty deeds." David knew that the only way he could give thanks in all circumstances was to focus on God and not on outer happenings. When we remember who God is and what He has done for us, we cannot help but join David in songs of thankfulness.

This week, we have looked at the appropriate response to God's love, mercy and compassion. Today it is time to express our thankfulness for the First Place program, which has made a lifestyle of thankfulness possible.

Turn back to week eight, Day 2. Using the words of Titus 3:3-8 as a guide, you were asked to write a summary. Copy your words in the following appropriate categories. Add any new thoughts that come to mind.

How it was

What happened

How life is now

Using these words and the lessons learned in this Bible study, compose a short essay on why you are thankful for First Place. Include the Scripture verses that are the cornerstone of your lifestyle of thankfulness. Also, be sure to list at least one reason why you are thankful for each of the Nine Commitments. Finally, list why you are thankful for an opportunity to study these lessons on thankfulness. You will be sharing your words with your First Place group during your victory celebration. Your presentation to the group should last about three minutes, so be concise.

*I am thankful for First Place because* . . .

"You are my God, and I will give you thanks; you are my God, and I will exalt you" (Psalm 118:28).

O Lord, I remember the days gone by; I meditate on all the works of Your hands in my life. I spread out my hands to You in thanksgiving (see Psalm 143:5-6).

# DAY SIX: *Reflections*

"This is the day that the LORD has made; let us rejoice and be glad in it" (Psalm 118:24). Today we are going to spend our time of reflection enjoying God's creation. Leave your books, pens and pencils behind and take a nature walk. All you will need to bring is a small tote bag. As you walk, purposefully observe the little things along your path: a rock that reminds you that God is your rock, a piece of wood that reminds you of the cross on which Jesus died for you, a dry leaf that exhorts you not to be disconnected from the vine, a pinecone that tells you new life comes from fallen things. Collect at least 10 small items to bring home with you. If you find a "postcard" from God that is too large to put in your bag, stop and thank God for giving you that special reminder that He cares for you. Make it your goal to find at least 25 reasons to be thankful as you enjoy this day God that has made for your pleasure. Use the things you normally overlook as reminders to rejoice in His compassion, mercy and love. Celebrating God in nature is one of the many benefits of living a life characterized by thankfulness.

The earth is Yours, O Lord, and You created everything in it. Help me to appreciate the beauty of Your wonderful creation that so clearly displays the works of Your hands (see Psalm 24:1).

Thank You, gracious Father, for giving me reminders of just how much You love me. Everywhere I look, I see Your footprints.

Lord Jesus, while on Earth You used common, everyday aspects of nature to teach great spiritual truths. Teach me about You from the everyday things of my life as well.

# DAY SEVEN: *Reflections*

The apostle Paul was a man who knew trial and tribulation; yet he had learned to be content in whatever circumstances the Lord orchestrated. Even in the midst of persecution, shipwreck, imprisonments and betrayal, Paul couldn't help but break forth in great benedictions that expressed the thankfulness that overtook his heart in every circumstance he faced.

It seems fitting to end this Bible study on the topic of thankfulness with one such benediction. Perhaps you would like to read it aloud in thankful celebration. In so doing, you would join saints throughout the ages who expressed the incredible richness of God's love that allowed them to give thanks in all things. Let this prayer, found in Ephesians 3:14-21, be Paul's prayer for you.

> I kneel before the Father, from whom his whole family in heaven and on earth derives its name. I pray that out of his glorious riches he may strengthen you with power through his Spirit in your inner being, so that Christ may dwell in your hearts through faith. And I pray that you, being rooted and established in love, may have power, together with all the saints, to grasp how wide and long and high and deep is the love of Christ, and to know this love that surpasses knowledge—that you may be filled to the measure of all the fullness of God. Now to him who is able to do immeasurably more than all we ask or imagine, according to his power that is at work within us, to him be glory in the church and in Christ Jesus throughout all generations, for ever and ever! Amen.

# Group Prayer Requests   Today's Date:_____

| Name | Request | Results |
|------|---------|---------|
|      |         |         |
|      |         |         |
|      |         |         |
|      |         |         |
|      |         |         |
|      |         |         |
|      |         |         |
|      |         |         |
|      |         |         |
|      |         |         |
|      |         |         |
|      |         |         |
|      |         |         |
|      |         |         |

# CREATING A THANKFULNESS JOURNAL

*O Lord my God, I will give you thanks forever.*
Psalm 30:12

One of the easiest ways to foster an attitude of thankfulness is to create a thankfulness journal: a separate place to record those simple, everyday things for which we are grateful. Even though we already make daily entries in a prayer journal or spiritual diary, keeping a thankfulness journal is an essential exercise in developing a heart that gives thanks in all circumstances. Unlike other forms of journal writing, a thankfulness journal is for the explicit purpose of recording the things for which we are thankful. It serves as both an acknowledgement of what God has done for us and a daily challenge to recognize things for which we can be thankful, even on bad days.

Perhaps keeping a written list of "what I am thankful for today" seems too simplistic to be effective. Yet study after study has proven the positive impact of maintaining a thankfulness journal. Researchers have discovered that those who keep thankfulness journals on a daily basis also exercise more regularly, have fewer health problems, make greater progress toward important personal goals, experience less depression, handle stress more effectively, and have more energy and vitality. They even sleep better at night![1] Spiritual masters throughout the ages have maintained that those with thankful hearts reap God's choicest blessings. Isn't it amazing that something as simple as keeping a thankfulness journal can change the quality of life so drastically?

Another plus is that keeping a thankfulness journal is not only beneficial, but it is also fun! The remainder of this Wellness Worksheet will outline some basic steps that will help you get started on your thankfulness journal today.

## START IT NOW

Any kind of notebook will suffice for your thankfulness journal. The important thing is that your pages of gratitude are bound together and kept in a safe place rather than randomly scribbled on loose pieces of paper. Some people like to decorate the cover of their thankfulness journal; others like to draw pictures that describe the things and events for which they are thankful. A stationery store, arts and crafts retailer or scrapbook supply store will have ideas for customizing your journal. The more unique and personal the pages, the more likely you will be to visit the journal consistently. Most people find that they want enough space in their journals to record two or three month's worth of gratitude affirmations.

➤ Create your thankfulness journal and then complete the remainder of this Wellness Worksheet. Each section will give you an opportunity to begin filling the pages of your new outlet for thankfulness.

## KEEP IT SIMPLE

Unlike other spiritual journals, a thankfulness journal is not a place to process your feelings, cry out in lament or pour out your heart to God. The whole purpose of a thankfulness journal is to thank God for blessing you in ways too numerous to ever adequately recount. The pages of this journal will consist largely of one- to two-sentence statements beginning with "I am thankful for . . . " You can add drawings, mementos or small photographs to enrich your simple words. Try using colored pencils to add color and texture, or experiment with stickers or glitter. Your creativity is a precious gift from God that you are called to use in expressing your thankfulness to Him.

Place a Scripture heading at the top of each day's page to remind you exactly Who you are thanking. Searching the Scriptures for thankfulness verses each day and committing some of those verses to memory will play a key role in developing a lifestyle of thankfulness.

➤ As your first entry in your thankfulness journal, write a short statement expressing your thankfulness to God for a simple pleasure.

➤ Now draw a small picture next to your sentence that creatively expresses your gratitude.

# KEEP IT PRIVATE

This is your journal, with your personal thoughts, recorded for your benefit and God's glory. Keep it in a safe place. If you write thinking others might read your words, you will tend to write what you want them to hear. You can share thoughts with trusted others, but the pages of this sacred journal are intended for your eyes only. God, who sees what you write on these private pages, will reward you (see Matthew 6:6).

➤ Share a private thanksgiving with God in the pages of your thankfulness journal.

# KEEP IT HONEST

Only you and God are going to see what is written on these pages, so you have absolutely no reason to exaggerate, minimize or force your feelings. List only those things for which you are genuinely grateful. God knows your thoughts before you even write them on the page (see Psalm 139:4). This is not a place for pious platitudes or lofty idealism. Heartfelt gratitude is always about the truth as it applies to your life in the present moment.

➤ Write a thankfulness truth that applies to your life in the present moment.

# KEEP IT PERSONAL

Comparisons and judgments have no place in your thankfulness journal. This journal is about you and your relationship with God, not about your neighbors. Remember, the Pharisee whom Jesus criticized prayed, "God, I thank you that I am not like other men" (Luke 18:11). We never need to fill our cup of thankfulness by devaluing another human being or feeding our vain ego at another's expense. God is never pleased with such a phony show of gratitude. Gratitude is about giving God thanks for the wonderful things He has done for us, not telling Him what wonderful things we have done for Him.

➤ List one great thing that God has done for you that fills you with joy.

## KEEP IT SPECIFIC

Rather than writing generalized statements such as "I am thankful that God is faithful," write about a specific instance that reminded you of God's faithfulness. Perhaps you saw or heard something today that brought God's loving-kindness to memory. For example, rather than being thankful for the sun, write about how the sun touched your skin and brought warmth to your soul.

➤ What recent occurrence reminded you of God's loving-kindness? Write it down as a thank offering.

## KEEP IT GOD-AFFIRMING

We should only be grateful for sources of health and healing, never for anything that erodes our relationship with God, damages His creation or harms our neighbor. Likewise, we can never be truly thankful for anything that harms God's Holy Spirit, who resides in our hearts, or that destroys our body, His earthly temple (see 1 Corinthians 6:19-20). You can even use your thankfulness journal as a type of accountability partner. Ask yourself, *Is this something I can write about in my thankfulness journal?* If the answer is no, then it is not beneficial for you.

➤ Think of something you have done today that you cannot write about with thankfulness. Now, thank God that He forgives you for doing that specific thing.

## KEEP IT CONSISTENT

Make adding entries to your thankfulness journal a daily habit. Begin by writing down five simple pleasures for which you are thankful each morning when you first wake up. Before you go to bed that night, record another five things for which you are thankful. Five each morning, five each evening, seven days a week; perhaps you are thinking, *I couldn't possibly find*

*70 things to be thankful for each week!* Remember, we are *training* our minds to develop a lifestyle of thankfulness. We must fight the scarcity mentality that makes us fear that we will not have enough thankfulness to write 70 "I am thankful" sentences each week. Just write down five in the morning and five in the evening today and trust that there will be five in the morning and five in the evening again tomorrow.

➣ Although writing prayers in your thankfulness journal should not be normal practice, compose a prayer that expresses your commitment to keep your journal daily. Remember, when we commit our plans to the Lord, they will succeed (see Proverbs 16:3)!


## REVIEW IT OFTEN

Reread your thankfulness entries often, especially on the days when you need to be reminded of God's faithful love. On a day when life is dark and gloomy, you can begin your thankfulness entries by thanking God that He has given you the grace to keep a thankfulness journal to read! Once a month, carve out time to read all 280-plus entries that you made during the month and bask in the warmth of God's love and care. As you notice a gradual shift in your outlook and attitude, be sure to thank God for that too. Each time you thank God, He will give you even more reasons to thank Him! You will be amazed at how God will bring health and healing as you faithfully practice giving Him thanks in all circumstances. God delights in those who delight in Him, and He showers them with His abundant blessings.

Note
1   Robert A. Emmons and Michael E. McCullough, "Highlights from the Research Project on Gratitude and Thankfulness." http://www.psy.miami.edu/faculty/mmccullough/gratitude/highlights_fall_2003.pdf (accessed April 6, 2005).

You are my God, and I will give you thanks;
you are my God, and I will exalt you.

Psalm 118:28

Date:

You are my God. This morning I give You thanks for:

1.

2.

3.

4.

5.

Tonight I am especially thankful for:

1.

2.

3.

4.

5.

# OVERFLOWING WITH THANKFULNESS

*I praise you because I am fearfully and wonderfully made;*
*your works are wonderful, I know that full well.*
Psalm 139:14

We can easily pay lip service to God for making us unique and special creations, but applying that concept to our lives is much more difficult. We tend to forget that our uniqueness is not limited to physical appearance, fingerprints and DNA. We receive, process and communicate information in our own unique and special styles, according to the gifts, talents and abilities that God has fashioned into our beings.

Expanding on the work of Howard Gardner, educators have discovered eight distinct ways people process and express information.[1] These are often referred to as "intelligence styles" or "learning styles," but they apply to all aspects of life—including how we express our thankfulness to God. This Wellness Worksheet will help you discover your unique thankfulness style—a style that reflects a facet of God's own image—and will give you an opportunity to express thankfulness in that way.

On the pages that follow, you will find brief descriptions of the eight thankfulness styles. As you read these descriptions, take note of which ones resonate in you and then experiment with the different suggestions listed for each thankfulness style. You will probably find two or three that fit you most and two or three that fit you least; the remaining styles will probably fall somewhere in the middle. Use the space in between the thankfulness styles for notes and thoughts. Once you discover the styles that fit you best, incorporate them into your lifestyle of thankfulness.

## VERBAL-LINGUISTIC

*I will extol the LORD at all times; his praise will always be on my lips.*
Psalm 34:1

## Strengths

- Has a natural ability to use words and language
- Understands root meanings of words
- Presents material convincingly
- Makes a good speaker, writer, storyteller and teacher
- Expresses thoughts and emotions most naturally in words

## Thankfulness Ideas

- Write in a journal
- Write poems and prayers expressing thankfulness
- Tell stories that illustrate God's faithful love and foster thankfulness in others
- Use humor and wit to captivate listeners
- Give public testimony to God's goodness
- Tell others about First Place through written or verbal communication

**Notes**

# VISUAL-SPATIAL

*He makes me lie down in green pastures, he leads me beside quiet waters.*
Psalm 23:2

## Strengths

- Is able to create vivid mental images and then use color, texture and design to portray those images
- Excels at crafts and interior design
- Likes graphs and charts
- Expresses thoughts and emotions in images, colors and designs

## Thankfulness Ideas

- Use brightly colored pages in your thankfulness journal
- Visualize God's goodness and love and express it through art and design
- Map the thoughts in your mind rather than journaling
- Use stickers, fabric and pictures to express thankfulness
- Create special cards to share with others that give thanks to God through artistic expression

**Notes**

# LOGICAL-MATHEMATICAL

*"To whom will you compare me? Or who is my equal?" says the Holy One.*
Isaiah 40:25

## Strengths

- Understands logic and numbers
- Has the ability to reason through and connect pieces of information
- Is able to ask questions and reason through complex problems
- Expresses thoughts and emotions in concepts and sequences

## Thankfulness Ideas

- Create logical progression sequences that prove God's faithfulness
- Number your journal entries
- Recall chronology of events that led to thankfulness
- Use God's Word to solve complex problems
- Question and then affirm God's love
- Use reason to convince others of God's faithfulness and love

**Notes**

# Body-Kinesthetic

*For in him we live and move and have our being.*
Acts 17:28

## Strengths

- Is able to express thought and emotion through movement
- Possesses balance and eye-hand coordination
- Has keen body awareness
- Appreciates the gift of movement
- Expresses thoughts and emotions while in motion

## Thankfulness Ideas

- Mime Scripture
- Praise God while walking or exercising
- Feel God's pleasure while moving your body
- Dance and use hand motions and body language that express gratitude
- Lead your First Place group in a charades exercise that expresses God's enduring love and mighty power
- Use your body as a living expression of God's grace

**Notes**

# MUSICAL-RHYTHMIC

*Let us come before him with thanksgiving and extol him with music and song.*
Psalm 95:2

## Strengths

- Produces and appreciates music
- Enjoys praising God through song
- Understands rhythm and tonal patterns
- Can hear sounds others miss
- Can lead others in worship through music
- Expresses thoughts and emotions through sounds, rhythms and patterns

## Thankfulness Ideas

- Sing and whistle as you go about your day
- Compose praise songs
- Lead worship through music
- Move in rhythmic patterns
- Recite psalms using the rhythm built into these prayers
- Play musical instruments that give sounds of praise
- Share your gift of music with your First Place group so that they can also worship through music

**Notes**

# NATURALIST-ENVIRONMENTAL

*Holy, holy, holy is the LORD Almighty; the whole earth is full of his glory.*
Isaiah 6:3

## Strengths

- Has a profound love for animals, plants and nature
- Enjoys communion with the natural world
- Appreciates God's work of creation
- Is interested in ecology and conservation
- Expresses thoughts and emotions in terms of nature and creation

## Thankfulness Ideas

- Take nature walks and hikes through God's creation
- Connect naturally occurring objects with God's attributes
- Thank God by caring for His world
- Teach others about God's creation
- Take your First Place group on a scavenger hunt and help them see God's wonders in nature
- Stop and smell the roses, and teach others to do the same

**Notes**


# INTERPERSONAL

*How good and pleasant it is when brothers live together in unity!*
Psalm 133:1


## Strengths

- Has the ability to relate to and understand others
- Maintains peace in group settings
- Encourages others to join in communion
- Possesses great organizational skills
- Expresses thoughts and emotions in group settings

## Thankfulness Ideas

- Create a small group in order to pray and discuss thankfulness
- Share blessings with others through phone calls and personal visits
- Join or start a prayer-chain ministry in your church and First Place group
- Help with celebration gatherings
- Encourage others to join you in thankfulness
- Share your love of people with everyone you meet

**Notes**

# INTRAPERSONAL

*Find rest, O my soul, in God alone; my hope comes from him.*
Psalm 62:5

## Strengths

- Is self-reflective and aware
- Understands dreams, visions and process
- Enjoys silence and solitude
- Is able to grasp and think through spiritual truths
- Expresses thoughts and emotions through introspection

## Thankfulness Ideas

- Meditate on God and His goodness
- Reason within yourself to overcome doubts and fears
- Find discernment in stillness and silence
- Be still and allow God's goodness to resonate in your soul
- Practice contemplative prayer and teach others to do the same
- Share your gift of meditation with your First Place group

# Notes

≫ Which three thankfulness styles best fit you?

How can you combine these strengths to create a style of thankfulness that is uniquely your own?

≫ What can you do today to begin incorporating your unique style of thankfulness into your daily life?

**Note**

1. Adapted from Howard Gardner, *Intelligence Reframed: Multiple Intelligences for the 21st Century* (New York: Basic Books, 2000).

# LEADER'S DISCUSSION GUIDE

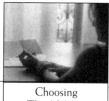

**Note:** As the leader of the group, complete Wellness Worksheet Two before the first group meeting. Once you understand the different thankfulness styles, you can find ways to include all eight styles in your lessons.

## Week One: Thankful for God's Enduring Love

1. **Before the meeting**: Make photocopies of Psalm 136 to ensure that the group will be reading from the same version. Begin the meeting by reading Psalm 136 responsively. Ask one or two people to lead by reading the first part of each praise statement. The group will then respond in unison, "His love endures forever."

2. The introduction to this week's lessons explained the secret to giving thanks in all circumstances. Ask several group members to paraphrase the words of Psalm 77:11-12 and to give an example of how this passage has been true in their lives.

3. Write "Slavery in Egypt" and "Enslavement to Food" at the top of a whiteboard or poster board. Ask the group to describe the similarities and differences between these two types of oppression. Record the group's answers under the respective columns.

4. On Day 4, we looked up four New Testament passages that spoke of our victory in Jesus. Ask each member to share which of the four passages presently seems most relevant to his or her Christian walk and why it seems so relevant.

5. As a group, discuss how it could be possible for the Israelites to forget God's goodness just three days after He delivered them. Ask, **What can we do to ensure that we do not do likewise?**

6. Review the concept of euphoric recall as it applies to the First Place Live-It plan.

7. Ask the members to share the insights they gained this week about God's enduring love. Compile their answers on a whiteboard or poster board.

8. Ask each group member to select one of the affirmations of God's goodness they listed on Days 1 and 3. Go around the room and have each person proclaim God's goodness using one of his or her statements. After each affirmation, have the group respond in unison, "Give thanks to the LORD, for he is good. His love endures forever" (Psalm 136:1). You may go around the room more than once if time permits!

# Week Two: Thankful for God's Strength

1. Ask volunteers to read Genesis 17:1, Genesis 35:11, Exodus 3:15 and Exodus 6:2-3. Lead a discussion on how God reveals Himself to His people through the names He uses to describe Himself.

2. **Before the meeting**: Ask two or three members if they would be willing to share which of the eight benefits listed in Psalm 91:14-16 they need most right now.

   Read Psalm 91:14-16. See how many group members can identify all eight benefits listed in these three short verses. Be sure you have identified them yourself before the meeting! Ask the volunteers you selected before the meeting to share. Afterwards, lead the group in prayer, asking God to hear and grant their requests.

3. Write the names "Mary" and "Hannah" on a whiteboard or poster board. Ask the group to share what these two women had in common. Focus on their common bond of thankfulness in adversity. Ask one person to record the group's answers on the board.

4. Paul and Silas sang hymns in prison and the other prisoners listened. Lead a discussion about how songs of thanksgiving open the ears of unbelievers when a more aggressive form of evangelism might close them.

5. Ask each group member to identify one way in which his or her weakness gives God an opportunity to display His strength.

6. Read Psalm 13 and ask the group to identify how praise and lament are woven together in this psalm. Remind the group that the book of Psalms contains many wonderful examples of the full range of human emotions that we can express to God in prayer.

7.  On a whiteboard or poster board, compile a list of all the great things God has done in and through the group members because of the First Place program.

8.  To close the meeting, have each person offer a short prayer in anticipation of blessing, thanking God in advance for granting his or her requests.

# Week Three: Thankful for God's Compassionate Care

1.  Write the words "Careless Shepherd" and "Unfortunate Sheep" on a whiteboard or poster board. Using the lists the group members compiled on Day 1, brainstorm the characteristics of each category.

2.  Discuss the differences between how God delivered the Israelites from bondage in Egypt and His actions in Ezekiel 34:11-16. In the course of the discussion, ask members to identify anything new they learned about God during this assignment.

3.  Discuss how the sheep's abuse of each other was a direct reflection of the shepherd's neglect. Ask the group to share what they learned about the need for loving discipline and a shepherd who models caring, compassionate love to his flock. How does this lesson apply to the churches the group members attend?

4.  Have a volunteer read Galatians 5:13-26. Focusing specifically on verses 14 and 15, ask the group to identify what God admonished the Galatians to do and the consequences if they failed to heed His words.

5.  **Before the meeting**: Ask one or two members to share a diet horror story that illustrates how we can be duped into doing things that harm us by people eager to make money off our misfortune.

    Have these group members share their stories at this time.

6.  **Before the meeting**: Write sequential numbers on small pieces of paper, one for each group member.

    Have each member draw a number at this time. Beginning with number one, have each member give a brief encouragement that expresses care and compassion to the person with the next sequential number. The last person will affirm the member who began the exercise.

7. Day 6 may have brought up a variety of emotions for the group members. Discuss how our former ways of life have been changed through our participation in First Place. Perhaps one or two members would be willing to share the drawings they made depicting the mess they left behind when they came to First Place.

8. Close the meeting with prayer, thanking God for His compassionate care of each group member.

## Week Four: Thankful for God's Guidance

1. Ask a group member to read John 10:1-18 out loud. Ask volunteers to share what it means to them personally that Jesus knows them intimately and calls them to follow Him.

2. Drawing from the details of Zacchaeus's story, ask group members to describe creative ways they have overcome the obstacles that kept them from actively seeking Jesus and how First Place is part of that journey.

3. We all have reservations about wholeheartedly following Jesus. Share your own fears and then invite others in the group to share their fears. If you still partially fear giving up a disordered relationship with food, be transparent about that aspect of your life.

4. Abandonment is one of the most primal human fears. It goes back to the time when, as infants, we were totally dependent on our caregivers for survival. Lead a discussion on how a personal relationship with the living God is the solution to that universal fear.

5. One of the Holy Spirit's many roles is to convict us of sin. Ask two or three group members to share how the Spirit's conviction brought them to the First Place program.

6. Discuss the different meanings of the Greek word "paracletos." As each meaning is given, have someone share how the Holy Spirit has played that role in his or her life.

7. End the meeting with prayer, thanking God for His guidance and for His promise to never forsake us or fail us.

## Week Five: Thankful for the Privilege of Prayer

1. Ask volunteers to repeat all five memory verses. Award each volunteer

with a gold star sticker to put in his or her thankfulness journal or with some other small prize.

2. Label a whiteboard or poster board with the following references: 1 Kings 8:30, Nehemiah 1:6 and Daniel 9:17. Ask the group to identify and discuss at least three common threads found among these prayers.

3. Prayer is meant to be a passionate expression of our love for God. Ask a volunteer to read Psalm 61 with expression that shows the emotion of this psalm. Ask several group members to share times when they were at the end of their ropes and cried out to God for relief and how God led them to a high rock of shelter.

4. Talk about the importance of dwelling in God's tent forever, rather than running to God only in times of need and then going our own way when the trouble has subsided.

5. We have a wonderful heritage as children of God. Ask the group to list some of the benefits of being part of God's family. Be sure the privilege of prayer is on that list!

6. Equate the First Place program commitments to fulfilling our vows day after day. Ask members to share how diligently keeping the Nine Commitments is part of our praise and thanksgiving to God.

7. To illustrate the concept of word bridges, have members describe the thoughts, feelings and emotions that the word "fun" evokes. Ask each member to share which of the four Day 7 images evoked the strongest emotions and why.

8. Close the meeting by reading Psalm 66:20 in unison, followed by a time of prayer.

## Week Six: Thankful for Dark Days

1. Ask group members whether they are keeping thankfulness journals. Ask one or two members who are doing so to share the benefits they have derived from the practice of observing God's simple blessings.

2. Read James 1:2-8 as a group. Discuss the dangers of basing our faith on feelings. Be sure to talk about James's illustration of an anchorless ship being tossed about by the waves. Ask, **How can God's precious promises serve as our anchor in troubling times?** Relate this discussion to the memory verse commitment of First Place.

3. Temptation is an opportunity to make a right choice. Ask members how this fact might change their thoughts and feelings about temptation.

4. Discuss why faithfulness to the First Place program gives witness to our profession of faith in God.

5. On Day 3, one of the descriptions given for God is that of a mother hen. Ask members to share the thoughts, feelings and images this picture of God evokes.

6. Read 1 Corinthians 11:31-32 as a group. Discuss how First Place is part of the self-discipline that keeps God from having to discipline us with sterner measures.

7. Ask members to share the insights they gained from the reflections on Days 6 and 7 and how they can use these insights as part of their lifestyles of thankfulness.

8. End the meeting with prayer, thanking God for being with us in dark days and for giving us rainbows and sunrises to remind us of His faithfulness and love.

## Week Seven: Thankful for God's Word

1. Ask a group member to read 2 Peter 3:1-2 as if he or she were reading a letter from a friend who is temporarily absent from the group. Ask each member of the group to describe the person most instrumental in bringing God's Word to him or her in a meaningful way.

2. On a whiteboard or poster board, list the different types of people that God uses to bring His Word into the lives of His disciples: proclaimers, encouragers, instructors, leaders and storytellers. Ask the group to identify well-known people who fit into one of the categories and who bring God's message of salvation through Jesus Christ. For example, Billy Graham is a proclaimer with whom we are all familiar.

3. Encouragement is one of the Nine Commitments of First Place. Ask members how they can incorporate God's Word into the encouragement they give to one another.

4. Priscilla and Aquila invited Apollos into their home and instructed him in the truth. Discuss how they handled Apollos's lack of information and what we can learn from their example.

5.  Write "Riches" and "God's Statutes" on a whiteboard or poster board. Compare the world's view of these ideals with the Christian view. How are they different? How are they similar?

6.  **Before the meeting**: Choose a good storyteller in the group and ask him or her to pick a favorite Bible story to tell the class.

    After the story, discuss how Bible stories have important lessons for children but also have a deeper application for adult listeners.

7.  Ask each group member to identify which type of servant from this week's lesson best describes him or her: proclaimer, encourager, instructor, leader or storyteller.

8.  Close in prayer, asking God to bless those He uses to bring His Word into the lives of others.

## Week Eight: Thankful for God's Grace

1.  Have a musically inclined member lead the group in the first verse of "Amazing Grace." The words are printed at the beginning of Day 1.

2.  Ask two or three volunteers to share with the group what it was like before they found First Place.

3.  Discuss the implications of the quote from Augustine: "God loves each of us as if there were only one of us." Share the depth of your gratitude when you realized Jesus went to the cross for you personally and then invite others to do the same.

4.  Discuss the difference between justification and sanctification. If you aren't clear on these two terms yourself, get your pastor or a spiritual mentor to explain them thoroughly before you lead this discussion.

5.  Ask members why grace must be accepted as a free gift.

6.  Talk about the benefits of both physical workouts and spiritual workouts.

7.  Copy the G.R.A.C.E. acrostic onto a whiteboard or poster board. Have members recall what word each letter represents and ask the group to share how this acrostic helps them understand the meaning of grace.

8.  During Day 7, we looked at the concept of balance. Discuss how putting Christ first in all things gives us balance in all four areas of our lives.

9. End this meeting by singing the last stanza of "Amazing Grace." It is printed at the end of Day 7.

## Week Nine: Thankful for Eternal Hope

1. Begin the meeting by reading the fill-in-the-blank sentences at the end of the introduction. Have the members say the missing words aloud as you read each sentence.

2. Discuss the importance of being fit to occupy the place Jesus is preparing for us and how First Place is part of that preparation process.

3. John had a vision while exiled on the island of Patmos. Brainstorm what that experience might have been like for the beloved apostle. Ask members whether they would be willing to boldly speak the Word if they might be exiled for doing so.

4. The book of Revelation can be confusing because of its symbolism, yet it contains an important message for all believers. Read chapters 2 and 3 to the group and then discuss how the message to each church also applies to us.

5. Discuss the importance of receiving a letter from the Trinity, as we learned in Day 3. Read the fill-in-the-blank dedication and emphasize the importance of Christ's work that gives us our eternal hope.

6. Discuss how godly correction leads to repentance. How is First Place part of God's correction?

7. The "If . . . , then . . . " exercise on Day 6 may have been new to many members. Review this exercise carefully and be prepared to answer any questions group members may have about the difference between propositions and promises.

8. End the meeting by reading Psalm 100 while sitting, kneeling, standing and marching. Be sensitive to any physical limitations the group members might have. Before members leave, remind them to be prepared to share their First Place story at next week's meeting.

## Week Ten: A Lifestyle of Thankfulness

1. Talk briefly about choice and contentment, but move quickly into the testimony part of the meeting.

2. Be sure the group understands that each presentation will only last three minutes (use a timer if necessary). In that time, have members tell the abbreviated version of their First Place story. Remind members not to spend too much time on how it was, or they will never get to what happened and how life is now. After each testimony, briefly pray for that person.

3. End the meeting with Paul's benediction prayer (Ephesians 3:14-21), printed at the end of Day 7. If you have a powerful proclaimer in your group, ask him or her to pronounce this benediction over your group. Exhort the members to receive these words as personal prayers for their lives as they continue to live lifestyles of thankfulness.

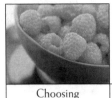

# FIRST PLACE
# MENU PLANS

*Each plan is based on approximately 1,400 calories.*

| | |
|---|---|
| Breakfast | 0-1 meats, 1-2 breads, 1 fruit, 0-1 milk, 0-½ fat |
| Lunch | 1-2 meats, 2 breads, 1 vegetable, 1 fruit, 1 fat |
| Dinner | 2-3 meats, 2 breads, 2 vegetables, 1 fat |
| Snacks | 1-2 breads, 1 fruit, 1 milk, ½-1 fat (or any remaining exchanges) |
| Daily Total | 4-5 meats, 6-7 breads, 3-4 vegetables, 3-4 fruits, 2-3 milks, 3-4 fats |

**Note**: You may always choose the high range for vegetables and fruits, but limit high range to only one category in meats, breads, milks or fats.

*For more calories, add the following to the 1,400-calorie plan:*

| | |
|---|---|
| 1,600 calories | 2 breads, 1 fat |
| 1,800 calories | 2 meats, 3 breads, 1 vegetable, 1 fat |
| 2,000 calories | 2 meats, 4 breads, 1 vegetable, 3 fats |
| 2,200 calories | 2 meats, 5 breads, 1 vegetable, 1 fruit, 5 fats |
| 2,400 calories | 2 meats, 6 breads, 2 vegetables, 1 fruit, 6 fats |

The exchanges for these meals were calculated using the MasterCook software. It uses a database of over 6,000 food items prepared using United States Department of Agriculture (USDA) publications and information from food manufacturers. As with any nutritional program, MasterCook calculates the nutritional values of the recipes based on ingredients. Nutrition may vary due to how the food is prepared, where the food comes from, soil content, season, ripeners, processing and methods of preparation. For these reasons, please use the recipes and menu plans as approximate guides. As always, consult your physician and/or a registered dietitian before starting a diet program.

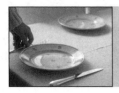

**Note:** We've included bonus recipes in this study's menu plans. Recipes for *italicized* items in menus can be found in each mealtime section.

## 🍎 Breakfast

2 slices whole-wheat bread, toasted; topped with
1 egg, cooked in a nonstick pan; and
1 strip turkey bacon, cooked crisp
1 medium apple

**Exchanges: 2 meats, 2 breads, 1 fruit, 1 fat**

~~~~~~~~~~~~~~~~~~~~~~~~~~~~~~~~~~~~~~~~~~~~~~~~~~~~

¾ c. Rice Chex cereal
½ English muffin
1 tsp. all-fruit spread
1 c. nonfat milk
½ medium banana

**Exchanges: 2 breads, 1 fruit, 1 milk**

~~~~~~~~~~~~~~~~~~~~~~~~~~~~~~~~~~~~~~~~~~~~~~~~~~~~

3 4-in. low-fat pancakes
1 tbsp. sugar-free syrup
1 c. strawberries, sliced
1 c. nonfat milk

**Exchanges: 2 breads, 1 fruit, 1 milk, ½ fat**

~~~~~~~~~~~~~~~~~~~~~~~~~~~~~~~~~~~~~~~~~~~~~~~~~~~~

½ c. cooked grits
1 tsp. reduced-fat margarine
1 slice diet whole-wheat bread, toasted
1 tsp. all-fruit spread
1 small banana
1 c. nonfat milk

**Exchanges: 2 breads, 1 fruit, 1 milk, ½ fat**

~~~~~~~~~~~~~~~~~~~~~~~~~~~~~~~~~~~~~~~~~~~~~~~~~~~~

1  *Oatmeal-Blueberry Muffin*
1  medium fresh peach
1  c. artificially sweetened nonfat yogurt
**Exchanges: 2 breads, 1 fruit, 1 milk, 1 fat**

~~~~~~~~~~~~~~~~~~~~~~~~~~~~~~~~~~~~~~~~~~~~~~~~~~~~~~~~~

1  3-in. canned biscuit, baked
1  tsp. all-fruit spread
½  medium banana
1  c. nonfat milk
**Exchanges: 1 bread, 1 fruit, 1 milk, 1 fat**

~~~~~~~~~~~~~~~~~~~~~~~~~~~~~~~~~~~~~~~~~~~~~~~~~~~~~~~~~

**Breakfast Delight**
Alternate the following ingredients in a parfait dish:
1  1½-in. square graham cracker, crumbled
8  oz. artificially sweetened nonfat yogurt
4  walnut halves, chopped
½  c. strawberries, sliced, or ½ c. blueberries
3  tbsp. wheat germ or 2 tbsp. bran cereal
**Exchanges: 2 breads, 1 fruit, 1 milk, 1 fat**

~~~~~~~~~~~~~~~~~~~~~~~~~~~~~~~~~~~~~~~~~~~~~~~~~~~~~~~~~

½  small (2 oz.) whole-wheat bagel
1  tsp. peanut butter
1  tsp. all-fruit spread
¾  c. Special K cereal
1  small banana
1  c. nonfat milk
**Exchanges: 2 breads, 1 fruit, 1 milk, 1 fat**

~~~~~~~~~~~~~~~~~~~~~~~~~~~~~~~~~~~~~~~~~~~~~~~~~~~~~~~~~

1  McDonald's Egg McMuffin
6  oz. orange juice
**Exchanges: 2 meats, 2 breads, 1 fruit, 1 fat**

~~~~~~~~~~~~~~~~~~~~~~~~~~~~~~~~~~~~~~~~~~~~~~~~~~~~~~~~~

*Cottage Cheese Omelet*
1  c. strawberries
*Banana Smoothie*
**Exchanges: 1 meat, 1 fruit, 1 milk, ½ fat**

~~~~~~~~~~~~~~~~~~~~~~~~~~~~~~~~~~~~~~~~~~~~~~~~~~~~~~~~~

½ large (4 oz.) whole-wheat bagel, toasted

2 tbsp. nonfat cream cheese

1 small orange

1 c. nonfat milk

Exchanges: ½ meat, 2 breads, 1 fruit, 1 milk

~~~~~~~~~~~~~~~~~~~~~~~~~~~~~~~~~~~~~~~~~~~~~~~~~~~

1 slice cinnamon-raisin bread, toasted

1 tsp. reduced-calorie margarine

½ tsp. granulated sugar

Pinch cinnamon

¾ c. plain nonfat yogurt

¾ c. blueberries

Exchanges: 1½ breads, 1 fruit, 1 milk, ½ fat

~~~~~~~~~~~~~~~~~~~~~~~~~~~~~~~~~~~~~~~~~~~~~~~~~~~

2 slices diet whole-wheat bread, toasted

1 tbsp. low-fat peanut butter

½ medium grapefruit

1 c. nonfat milk

Exchanges: ½ meat, 1 bread, ½ fruit, 1 milk, ½ fat

~~~~~~~~~~~~~~~~~~~~~~~~~~~~~~~~~~~~~~~~~~~~~~~~~~~

2 low-fat frozen waffles, heated

1 tsp. reduced-calorie margarine

2 tsp. sugar-free syrup

½ small mango

1 c. nonfat milk

Exchanges: 2 breads, 1 fruit, 1 milk, ½ fat

## BONUS BREAKFAST RECIPES

### *Banana Smoothie*

⅓ c. nonfat powdered milk

2 tsp. cocoa

½ medium banana, mashed

1  c. water
4  ice cubes

Mix all ingredients in blender and serve immediately. Serves 1.
**Exchanges: 1 fruit, 1 milk**

**Note**: You can vary the recipe with different fruits ($\frac{3}{4}$ c. strawberries, blueberries, etc.). You can also freeze this recipe to eat rather than drink.

~~~~~~~~~~~~~~~~~~~~~~~~~~~~~~~~~~~~~~~~~~~~~~~~~~~~

## Cottage Cheese Omelet

1  egg
2  egg whites
1  tbsp. water
1  tsp. dried parsley flakes
$\frac{1}{2}$  tsp. salt
$\frac{1}{4}$  tsp. dried whole marjoram
$\frac{1}{4}$  tsp. black pepper
1  oz. low-fat cottage cheese
   Nonstick cooking spray

Combine egg, egg whites, water and seasonings in a small bowl; stir well. Coat a medium-size nonstick skillet with nonstick cooking spray; place over medium heat until hot enough to make a drop of water sizzle. Pour egg mixture into pan. As egg mixture starts to cook, gently lift edges of omelet with a spatula and tilt pan to force uncooked portion to flow underneath. When egg mixture is almost set, spoon cottage cheese over half of omelet; continue cooking until egg mixture is set. Loosen omelet with a spatula and fold in half; slide onto serving platter and serve immediately. Serves 2.
**Exchanges: 1 meat, $\frac{1}{2}$ fat**

~~~~~~~~~~~~~~~~~~~~~~~~~~~~~~~~~~~~~~~~~~~~~~~~~~~~

# Oatmeal-Blueberry Muffins

  1  c. plus 2 tbsp. all-purpose flour
  6  oz. uncooked rolled oats
  1  tbsp. baking powder
      Sugar substitute to equal 2 tbsp. sugar
 ½  tsp. salt
  1  c. nonfat milk
  1  egg
 ¼  c. vegetable oil
  1  c. fresh blueberries
  1  tsp. ground cinnamon
      Nonstick cooking spray

Preheat oven to 425° F. In a medium bowl, combine flour, oats, baking powder, sugar substitute and salt; make a well in center of mixture. Combine milk, egg and oil; add to dry ingredients, stirring just until moistened. Gently fold in blueberries. Spoon batter into muffin pans coated with nonstick cooking spray, filling two-thirds full. Sprinkle cinnamon over muffins. Bake 20-25 minutes or until lightly browned. Serves 12.

**Exchanges: 1 bread, 1 fat**

## ☙ LUNCH

# Beef Stir-Fry

  1  lb. lean boneless top-round steak, trimmed
 ⅔  c. water
 ¼  c. chopped onion
  3  tbsp. reduced-sodium soy sauce
  1  tsp. beef-flavored bouillon granules
  1  tsp. Worcestershire sauce
  1  clove garlic, minced
 ½  tsp. salt
 ⅛  tsp. pepper
  2  medium carrots, peeled and sliced diagonally

2 c. cauliflower flowerets
1 c. sliced fresh mushrooms
1 6-oz. pkg. frozen snow peas, partially thawed
$\frac{1}{4}$ c. water
1 tbsp. cornstarch
Nonstick cooking spray

Partially freeze steak; slice diagonally across grain into $\frac{1}{4}$-inch strips; set aside. Combine water, onion, soy sauce, bouillon granules, Worcestershire sauce, garlic, salt and pepper in a large bowl. Add steak; stir to coat. Cover and refrigerate 1 hour, stirring once. Drain steak, reserving marinade. Set steak aside. Cook carrots and cauliflower for 3 minutes in just enough boiling water to cover the vegetables; drain and set aside. Coat a wok or large skillet with nonstick cooking spray; preheat on medium-high heat for 2 minutes. Add steak; stir-fry 3 minutes. Add mushrooms; stir-fry 1 minute. Add snow peas, carrots and cauliflower; stir-fry 2 minutes more or until vegetables are crisp-tender. Combine reserved marinade, $\frac{1}{4}$ cup water and cornstarch; stir to blend. Pour over steak mixture and stir-fry until thick and bubbly. Serves 6.

**Serve with** $\frac{2}{3}$ cup cooked white rice.
**Exchanges: 2 meats, 2 breads, 2 vegetables**

~ ~ ~ ~ ~ ~ ~ ~ ~ ~ ~ ~ ~ ~ ~ ~ ~ ~ ~ ~ ~ ~ ~ ~ ~ ~ ~ ~ ~ ~ ~ ~ ~ ~ ~ ~ ~ ~ ~ ~ ~ ~ ~ ~ ~ ~ ~ ~

# Lo Mein Take-Out
2 c. Chinese beef or chicken lo mein
$\frac{1}{2}$ c. steamed vegetables
1 c. cubed pineapple
**Exchanges: 2 meats, 2 breads, 2 vegetables, 1 fruit, 1 fat**

~ ~ ~ ~ ~ ~ ~ ~ ~ ~ ~ ~ ~ ~ ~ ~ ~ ~ ~ ~ ~ ~ ~ ~ ~ ~ ~ ~ ~ ~ ~ ~ ~ ~ ~ ~ ~ ~ ~ ~ ~ ~ ~ ~ ~ ~ ~ ~

# Spinach-Mandarin Salad
4 c. fresh spinach leaves
2 c. cherry tomatoes
$1\frac{1}{2}$ c. cubed, cooked chicken breast, chilled
1 c. thinly sliced radishes
$\frac{1}{2}$ lb. fresh mushrooms, sliced
$\frac{1}{2}$ c. croutons

*Mandarin Dressing*

2   tbsp. sesame seeds, toasted

Wash spinach leaves thoroughly in cold water; remove and discard stems. Place spinach in a large bowl. Add tomatoes, chicken, radishes, mushrooms and croutons. Add *Mandarin Dressing* and toss salad gently. Garnish salad with sesame seeds and serve on chilled plates. Serves 5.

**Serve with** 4 crisp bread sticks (4 x 1½ inches).

**Exchanges: 2½ meats, 2 breads, 1½ vegetables, ½ fat**

~ ~ ~ ~ ~ ~ ~ ~ ~ ~ ~ ~ ~ ~ ~ ~ ~ ~ ~ ~ ~ ~ ~ ~ ~ ~ ~ ~ ~ ~ ~ ~ ~ ~ ~ ~ ~ ~ ~ ~ ~ ~ ~ ~ ~ ~ ~ ~

## Black Beans and Rice

1   16-oz. package dried black beans
1   medium green pepper, chopped
¼   c. chopped onion, divided
10   c. water, divided
2   cloves garlic, minced
½   tsp. dried whole oregano
¼   tsp. ground cumin
3   tbsp. vinegar
1   tsp. salt
3   c. hot cooked rice (cooked without salt or fat)

Wash beans. Combine beans, green pepper and 2 tablespoons onion in a large Dutch oven. Cover with 6 cups of water and let soak overnight. Add remaining 4 cups water to Dutch oven; cover and bring to a boil. Reduce heat and simmer 2½ hours or until beans are tender. Combine remaining 2 tbsp. onion, garlic, oregano and cumin in a small bowl; mash mixture, using a fork. Stir in vinegar. Add vinegar mixture and salt to beans. Simmer, uncovered, an additional 20 minutes. Serve over hot, cooked rice. Serves 6.

**Serve with** salad greens tossed with fat-free Italian dressing, and 1 cup *Fruit Salad.*

**Exchanges: 2 breads, 2 vegetables**

~ ~ ~ ~ ~ ~ ~ ~ ~ ~ ~ ~ ~ ~ ~ ~ ~ ~ ~ ~ ~ ~ ~ ~ ~ ~ ~ ~ ~ ~ ~ ~ ~ ~ ~ ~ ~ ~ ~ ~ ~ ~ ~ ~ ~ ~ ~ ~

## Chicken Alfredo

1 Lean Cuisine Chicken Alfredo

2 c. fresh spinach, tossed with

$\frac{1}{2}$ c. sliced mushrooms and

Fat-free Italian dressing

**Exchanges:** 1 $\frac{1}{2}$ meats, 2 breads, 2 vegetables, $\frac{1}{2}$ milk

~~~~~~~~~~~~~~~~~~~~~~~~~~~~~~~~~~~~~~~~~~~~~~~~~

## Turkey Salad

5 oz. cooked low-fat turkey, cut into $\frac{1}{2}$-in. strips

2 c. chopped fresh, washed spinach leaves

2 medium tomatoes, sliced

1 10$\frac{1}{2}$-oz. can asparagus spears, drained and chopped

2 hard-cooked eggs, chopped

1 green onion, chopped

$\frac{1}{4}$ c. plus 2 tbsp. fat-free Italian dressing

$\frac{1}{4}$ c. prepared mustard

Combine turkey, spinach, tomatoes, asparagus, eggs and green onion in a large bowl. Cover and refrigerate until thoroughly chilled. Combine Italian dressing and mustard until well blended. Pour over salad; toss gently to coat.

**Serve with** one 2-ounce slice French bread and 1 cup sliced strawberries tossed with 1 tablespoon poppy seed dressing.

**Exchanges:** 2 meats, 2 breads, 2 vegetables, 1 fruit, 1 fat

~~~~~~~~~~~~~~~~~~~~~~~~~~~~~~~~~~~~~~~~~~~~~~~~~

## Chicken Noodle Soup

1 c. canned chicken noodle soup

1 c. broccoli florets with

2 tbsp. fat-free ranch dressing

1 slice Velveeta Light cheese

8 low-fat saltines

1 2-in. wedge honeydew melon

**Exchanges:** 1 meat, 2 breads, 1 vegetable, 1 fruit, 1 fat

~~~~~~~~~~~~~~~~~~~~~~~~~~~~~~~~~~~~~~~~~~~~~~~~~

# Grilled Chicken Sandwich

1   Chic-fil-A Grilled Chicken Sandwich
1   side carrot and raisin salad
  **Serve with** 15 red grapes.
**Exchanges: 3 meats, 2 breads, 1 vegetable, 1 fruit, 1 fat**

~~~~~~~~~~~~~~~~~~~~~~~~~~~~~~~~~~~~~~~~~~~~~~~~~~~~~~~~~~~

# Quick Vegetable Soup

1   12-oz. can V-8 juice, regular or spicy
1   c. water
½   onion, chopped
2   stalks celery, chopped
1   carrot, sliced
1   16-oz. can green beans, undrained
  Anything from the list of vegetable exchanges

Combine all ingredients in a large pot and simmer for about one hour.
Serves 3.
  **Serve with** 12 saltine crackers and ⅔ cup *Fruit Medley*.
**Exchanges: 2 breads, 2 vegetables, 1 fruit**

~~~~~~~~~~~~~~~~~~~~~~~~~~~~~~~~~~~~~~~~~~~~~~~~~~~~~~~~~~~

# Cheese Quesadilla

1   Taco Bell cheese quesadilla
½   c. salsa mixed with
1   tbsp. fat-free sour cream
1   c. carrot sticks with
¼   c. fat-free Ranch dressing
**Exchanges: 1 ½ meats, 2 breads, 2 vegetables, 2 fats**

~~~~~~~~~~~~~~~~~~~~~~~~~~~~~~~~~~~~~~~~~~~~~~~~~~~~~~~~~~~

# Chicken Fajita

1 ½   oz. cooked chicken, shredded
¼   c. onion, diced
¼   c. bell pepper, diced
¼   c. salsa

1   tbsp. fat-free sour cream
1   10-in. low-fat flour tortilla
¼   oz. Colby cheese, shredded
    Nonstick cooking spray

In a skillet coated with nonstick cooking spray, sauté onions and peppers
for one minute; add chicken and heat thoroughly. In a small bowl, combine
salsa and sour cream; mix well. Fill tortilla with chicken; top with cheese.
Heat in microwave, if desired; serve with creamy salsa. Serves 1.

**Serve with** 1 cup canned reduced-sugar tropical mixed fruit.
**Exchanges: 2 meats, 2 breads, 1 ½ vegetables, 1 fruit, 1 fat**

~~~~~~~~~~~~~~~~~~~~~~~~~~~~~~~~~~~~~~~~~~~~~~~~~~~~~~~~~~~~

## Sliced-Egg Sandwich
2   slices diet whole-wheat bread
2   tsp. low-fat mayonnaise
1   hard-cooked egg, sliced
¼   c. watercress leaves
2   tomato slices

Spread mayonnaise over bread slices. Layer with hard-cooked egg slices,
watercress leaves and tomato.

**Serve with** ½ cup each carrot and celery sticks and a 3 x 2-inch
wedge of watermelon.
**Exchanges: 1 meat, 1 bread, 1 vegetable, 1 fruit, 1 fat**

~~~~~~~~~~~~~~~~~~~~~~~~~~~~~~~~~~~~~~~~~~~~~~~~~~~~~~~~~~~~

## Chef's Salad
8   c. coarsely chopped iceberg lettuce
1   c. thinly sliced radishes
2   green onions, sliced
⅓   c. *Thousand Island Dressing*
2   oz. cooked low-fat ham, chopped
2   oz. cooked low-fat turkey, chopped
2   oz. low-fat American cheese, diced
2   oz. low-fat Swiss cheese, diced

2   small tomatoes, chopped

1   hard-cooked egg, chopped

Combine lettuce, radishes and green onions in a large bowl. Cover and refrigerate until thoroughly chilled. Add *Thousand Island Dressing;* toss gently to coat. Top with ham, turkey, American and Swiss cheeses, tomatoes and egg. Serves 8.

**Serve with** 1 *Quick and Easy Roll.*

**Exchanges: 1 meat, 1 bread, 1 vegetable**

~~~~~~~~~~~~~~~~~~~~~~~~~~~~~~~~~~~~~~~~~~~~~~~~~~~~

## *Scallops Parmesan*

1 1/4   lb. bay scallops

2   tbsp. reduced-fat margarine

1   clove garlic, chopped

2   tbsp. lemon juice

1   28-oz. can diced Italian-style tomatoes, not drained

1/4   c. shredded Parmesan cheese

Over medium-high heat, melt margarine in a skillet. Sauté garlic and scallops for 3 to 4 minutes; add lemon juice. Set aside and keep warm. In a separate skillet, cook tomatoes for 5 to 10 minutes, until slightly reduced. Add scallops mixture to tomatoes and heat thoroughly. Top with Parmesan cheese. Serves 4.

**Serve each with** 1/2 cup cooked brown rice, 1 cup steamed broccoli and 1 small (1-ounce) dinner roll.

**Exchanges: 3 meats, 2 breads, 1 1/2 vegetables, 1 fat**

# BONUS LUNCH RECIPES

## *Fruit Medley*

1   c. water-packed pineapple chunks or tidbits

1   c. fresh orange slices

1   c. diced, unpeeled apple

1 c. canned, unsweetened, drained cherries

1 c. plain nonfat yogurt

Combine pineapple, orange slices, apple and cherries in a medium bowl. Gently fold in yogurt. Cover and refrigerate until thoroughly chilled. Serves 7.

**Exchange: 1 fruit**

~~~~~~~~~~~~~~~~~~~~~~~~~~~~~~~~~~~~~~~~~~~~~~~~~~~~~~~~~~~~

## Fruit Salad

$\frac{1}{2}$ c. pineapple juice

1 tbsp. cornstarch

1 pkg. sugar substitute (optional)

$\frac{3}{4}$ c. pineapple chunks

1 small banana, peeled and sliced

1 kiwi, peeled and sliced

1 c. strawberries, sliced

1 small apple, cored and diced

Thicken pineapple juice with cornstarch in a saucepan over medium heat. (**Tip:** Mix the cornstarch with a little bit of water before adding to the juice so it won't be lumpy.) Cool; add sugar substitute, if desired. In a medium bowl, combine pineapple, banana, kiwi, strawberries and apple. Coat with thickened pineapple juice. Serves 6.

**Exchange: 1 fruit**

~~~~~~~~~~~~~~~~~~~~~~~~~~~~~~~~~~~~~~~~~~~~~~~~~~~~~~~~~~~~

## Mandarin Dressing

$\frac{1}{4}$ c. low-fat Italian dressing

2 tbsp. reduced-sodium soy sauce

1 tsp. vinegar

1 tsp. sesame seeds

Sugar substitute to equal 2 tbsp. sugar

$\frac{1}{8}$ tsp. pepper

Combine all ingredients in a jar; cover tightly and shake vigorously. Refrigerate at least 2 hours to blend flavors. Yields $\frac{1}{4}$ cup plus 2 tablespoons.

**Exchange: Free (serving size: 2 tablespoons)**

## Quick and Easy Rolls

2   c. self-rising flour
$\frac{1}{4}$   c. plus 2 tbsp. low-fat mayonnaise
1   c. nonfat buttermilk
    Nonstick cooking spray

Preheat oven to 375° F. Combine flour, mayonnaise and buttermilk; stir just until moistened. Spoon batter into muffin pans coated with nonstick cooking spray. Bake 12 to 15 minutes or until lightly browned. Yields 1 dozen rolls.

**Exchange (per roll): 1 bread**

## Thousand Island Dressing

1   c. plain nonfat yogurt
$\frac{1}{4}$   c. nonfat buttermilk
1   tbsp. low-fat mayonnaise
1   tbsp. chopped dill pickle
1   tbsp. catsup
1   tsp. chopped fresh parsley
$\frac{1}{8}$   tsp. seasoned salt

Combine yogurt, buttermilk and mayonnaise in a small bowl. Stir in pickle, catsup, parsley and seasoned salt. Cover and refrigerate until thoroughly chilled. Serving size: 2 tablespoons.

**Exchange: $\frac{1}{2}$ fat (for 2 tablespoons; 1 tablespoon is free)**

## Pork Chops with Apples

4  4-oz. lean center-cut pork chops, trimmed
1  medium onion, chopped
1¼  c. water
1  tsp. chicken-flavored bouillon granules
¼  tsp. pepper
4  medium cooking apples, peeled and sliced
½  tsp. cinnamon
   Nonstick cooking spray

Brown pork chops and onion in a large skillet coated with nonstick cooking spray. In a small bowl, stir together water, bouillon and pepper, until bouillon is dissolved; add to skillet. Cover and bring to a boil. Reduce heat; simmer 20 minutes. Skim off fat. Add apple slices and cinnamon to skillet. Cover and simmer an additional 15 minutes. Transfer to a serving platter and serve hot. Serves 4.

**Serve with** 1 cup mashed potatoes and 1 cup seasoned green beans.
Exchanges: 3 meats, 1 bread, 1 vegetable, 1 fruit
~~~~~~~~~~~~~~~~~~~~~~~~~~~~~~~~~~~~~~~~~~~~~~~~~~~~~

## Beef Burrito

1  Taco Bell Beef Burrito
1  Green salad with salsa and reduced-fat sour cream
1  c. carrot sticks
½  c. fresh pineapple, cubed
Exchanges: 2 meats, 3 breads, 1 vegetable, 1 fruit, 1 fat
~~~~~~~~~~~~~~~~~~~~~~~~~~~~~~~~~~~~~~~~~~~~~~~~~~~~~

## Pot Roast with Vegetables

1  lb. lean boneless chuck roast, trimmed
2  medium onions, peeled and sliced
4  stalks celery, sliced
¼  c. water

$\frac{1}{4}$  tsp. salt

 $\frac{1}{8}$  tsp. pepper

 6  large carrots, peeled and sliced

 4  medium red potatoes, peeled and coarsely chopped

Nonstick cooking spray

Preheat oven to 350° F. In a Dutch oven coated with nonstick cooking spray, brown chuck roast evenly on all sides over medium heat. Add sliced onion, celery, water, salt and pepper. Cover Dutch oven, place in oven and bake 1 hour and 15 minutes. Add carrots and potatoes; continue to bake, covered, for 1 hour or until meat and vegetables are tender. Transfer roast and vegetables to a serving platter; cut roast into 2-ounce slices. Serves 6.

**Serve with** 1 serving *Mexican Cornbread.*

**Exchanges: 2 meats, 2 breads, 1 vegetable, 1 fat**

~~~~~~~~~~~~~~~~~~~~~~~~~~~~~~~~~~~~~~~~~~~~~~~~~~~

## Six-Layer Dinner

 1  lb. lean ground chuck

 4  medium red potatoes, peeled and cut into $\frac{1}{4}$-in. slices

 1  large onion, cut into $\frac{1}{4}$-in. slices

 4  large carrots, peeled and cut into $\frac{1}{4}$-in. slices

 1  medium green pepper, cut into $\frac{1}{4}$-in. slices

 1  16-oz. can whole tomatoes, drained and chopped

 $\frac{1}{4}$  tsp. pepper

 $\frac{1}{8}$  tsp. dried basil

Preheat oven to 350° F. Cook ground chuck in a large ovenproof skillet with lid over medium heat until meat is browned, stirring to crumble. Pour meat into a colander and pat meat dry with paper towels. Wipe skillet with a paper towel. Return ground chuck to skillet and layer potatoes, onion, carrots, green pepper and tomatoes on top. Sprinkle with pepper and basil. Cover and bake 45 minutes. Serves 4.

**Serve with** 1 cup *Sautéed Greens.*

**Exchanges: 2 meats, 2 breads, 2 vegetables, 1 fat**

~~~~~~~~~~~~~~~~~~~~~~~~~~~~~~~~~~~~~~~~~~~~~~~~~~~

# Chicken Divan

 8   2½-oz. boneless, skinless chicken breast halves
 1   10-oz. pkg. frozen chopped broccoli
 ¼   10¾-oz. can cream of chicken soup
 ¼   10¾-oz. can cream of potato soup
 ½   c. nonfat milk
 1½   tsp. lemon juice
 2   tbsp. grated Parmesan cheese
    Nonstick cooking spray

Preheat oven to 350° F. Place chicken in a large saucepan and add just enough water to cover chicken. Cover and bring to a boil. Reduce heat; simmer 20 minutes or until chicken is cooked through; drain. Chop chicken and set aside. Cook broccoli according to package directions, omitting salt and fat; drain well. Arrange broccoli in a 2-quart baking dish coated with nonstick cooking spray; top with chicken. In a small bowl, combine soups, milk and lemon juice; pour over chicken and broccoli. Sprinkle with Parmesan cheese. Bake 25 minutes or until thoroughly heated. Serves 8.

**Serve with** 1 cup *Parmesan Peas* and 2 slices *Cheese Casserole Bread.*
**Exchanges: 2 meats, 2 breads, 2 vegetables, 2 fats**

~~~~~~~~~~~~~~~~~~~~~~~~~~~~~~~~~~~~~~~~~~~~~~~~~~~~~~~~~

# Stuffed Flounder Fillets

 4   2½ oz. flounder fillets
 ½   c. finely chopped onion
 1   clove garlic, minced
 ⅓   c. finely chopped celery
 ¼   c. finely chopped carrot
 ¼   c. minced sweet red pepper
 ⅛   tsp. ground thyme
 2   tbsp. chopped fresh parsley, divided
 1   tbsp. grated Parmesan cheese
 1   tbsp. low-fat mayonnaise
 ½   tsp. Dijon mustard
 1   tbsp. lemon juice
    Nonstick cooking spray

Preheat oven to 400° F. Rinse fillets thoroughly in cold water; pat dry with paper towels. Set aside. Coat a medium skillet with nonstick cooking spray; preheat over medium heat. Sauté onion and garlic until tender. Add celery, carrot and red pepper; cover and cook over medium-low heat, stirring occasionally, 5 minutes or until vegetables are tender. Stir in thyme; cook over medium-high heat until all moisture has evaporated. Stir in 1 tablespoon parsley. Spoon an equal amount of mixture in center of each fillet; roll up lengthwise and secure with a wooden pick. Place fish rolls, seam side down, in a shallow casserole dish coated with nonstick cooking spray. In a small bowl, combine Parmesan cheese, mayonnaise and mustard; spread mixture evenly over fish rolls. Sprinkle with lemon juice. Bake 20 minutes or until fish is lightly browned and flakes easily. Sprinkle with remaining 1 tablespoon parsley and serve. Serves 4.

**Serve with** 1 cup *Asparagus with Lemon Sauce* and one 2-ounce slice of French bread with 1 tablespoon reduced-fat margarine.

**Exchanges: 3 meats, 2 breads, 1 vegetable, 1 fat**

~ ~ ~ ~ ~ ~ ~ ~ ~ ~ ~ ~ ~ ~ ~ ~ ~ ~ ~ ~ ~ ~ ~ ~ ~ ~ ~ ~ ~ ~ ~ ~ ~ ~ ~ ~ ~ ~ ~ ~ ~ ~ ~ ~ ~ ~ ~ ~ ~

## Squash Mix with Chicken

| | |
|---|---|
| 1 | c. chopped, cooked chicken |
| 1 | c. chopped onion |
| 1 | c. sliced celery |
| 2 | tsp. reduced-fat margarine, melted |
| 5 | c. sliced yellow squash |
| 2 | c. sliced zucchini |
| 4 | tbsp. water |
| 1 | tsp. salt |
| 1 | tsp. dried whole chervil |
| $\frac{1}{4}$ | tsp. red pepper |
| $\frac{1}{4}$ | tsp. black pepper |

Sauté onion and celery in margarine in a large skillet until tender. Stir in squash and remaining ingredients. Cover and bring to a boil. Reduce heat; simmer 8 to 10 minutes or until vegetables are tender, stirring frequently. Transfer mixture to a serving dish; serve hot. Serves 4.

**Serve with** a 1-ounce dinner roll and 1 cup green salad with 2 table-spoons low-fat dressing.

Exchanges: 2 meats, 1 bread, 2 vegetables

~~~~~~~~~~~~~~~~~~~~~~~~~~~~~~~~~~~~~~~~~~~~~~~~~~~~~~

## Cheese Cannelloni

1   Stouffer's Lean Cuisine Cheese Cannelloni
1   1-oz. garlic breadstick
1   c. cooked green beans

Exchanges: 1 ½ meats, 2 ½ breads, 2 vegetables, 1 fat

~~~~~~~~~~~~~~~~~~~~~~~~~~~~~~~~~~~~~~~~~~~~~~~~~~~~~~

## Zucchini Quiche

1    tsp. cornstarch
¼    tsp. dried oregano
1    c. canned, stewed tomatoes, undrained
1 ½  c. nonfat milk
4    eggs
1    tbsp. flour
2    c. shredded zucchini
¼    c. chopped onion
½    c. shredded Swiss cheese
½    c. shredded low-fat American cheese
2    tbsp. grated Parmesan cheese
     Nonstick cooking spray

Preheat oven to 350° F. Combine cornstarch and oregano in a small sauce-pan. Add tomatoes and bring to a boil. Reduce heat; simmer 2 minutes or until thickened. Keep warm. Combine milk, eggs and flour in a large bowl; beat well, using a wire whisk. Add zucchini, onion and cheeses. Pour egg mixture into a 9-inch round quiche dish coated with nonstick cooking spray. Bake 1 hour. Spoon tomato mixture over quiche. Cut into wedges and serve warm. Serves 4.

**Serve with** 1 cup *Creamed Potato Soup* and one 2-ounce slice of Italian bread.

Exchanges: 2 meats, 2 breads, 2 vegetables, ½ fat

~~~~~~~~~~~~~~~~~~~~~~~~~~~~~~~~~~~~~~~~~~~~~~~~~~~~~~

# Baked Ham with Pineapple

  1  2-lb. fully cooked, boneless smoked ham
 20  whole cloves
  4  rings unsweetened canned pineapple, drained
 ½  c. diet ginger ale
  1  tsp. ground cinnamon

Preheat oven to 325° F. Remove and discard casing from ham. Score top of ham in a diamond design and stud with cloves. Place ham in a shallow baking dish and arrange pineapple slices over top. Pour ginger ale over ham and evenly sprinkle each pineapple slice with cinnamon. Bake 25 to 30 minutes, or until thoroughly heated. Serves 12.

    **Serve with** ⅔ cup roasted potatoes, 1 cup cooked green vegetables and a 1-ounce dinner roll topped with 1 teaspoon reduced-fat margarine. **Exchanges: 2 meats, 2 breads, 2 vegetables, 1 ½ fats**

~ ~ ~ ~ ~ ~ ~ ~ ~ ~ ~ ~ ~ ~ ~ ~ ~ ~ ~ ~ ~ ~ ~ ~ ~ ~ ~ ~ ~ ~ ~ ~ ~ ~ ~ ~ ~ ~ ~ ~ ~ ~ ~ ~ ~ ~ ~

# Chicken Dijon

  8  3-oz. chicken breast halves, skin removed
  4  oz. plain low-fat yogurt
 ¼  c. Dijon mustard
 ½  c. soft bread crumbs
    Nonstick cooking spray

Preheat oven to 450° F. Combine yogurt and mustard in a shallow bowl. Brush chicken breast halves with yogurt mixture, and then dredge in bread crumbs. Arrange chicken in a 12 x 8 x 2-inch baking dish coated with non-stick cooking spray. Cover and bake 30 minutes. Bake, uncovered, 15 minutes more, or until juices run pink and coating is browned. Serves 8.

    **Serve with** 1 cup *Marinated Garden Vegetables* and 1 cup cooked wild rice. **Exchanges: 2 meats, 1 bread, 2 vegetables**

~ ~ ~ ~ ~ ~ ~ ~ ~ ~ ~ ~ ~ ~ ~ ~ ~ ~ ~ ~ ~ ~ ~ ~ ~ ~ ~ ~ ~ ~ ~ ~ ~ ~ ~ ~ ~ ~ ~ ~ ~ ~ ~ ~ ~ ~ ~

# Pizza

  2  medium slices Pizza Hut Thin and Crispy Supreme
  1  tossed salad with

1 tbsp. low-fat salad dressing
1 c. sliced peaches
**Exchanges: 3 meats, 3 breads, 1 vegetable, 1 fruit, 2 fats**

~~~~~~~~~~~~~~~~~~~~~~~~~~~~~~~~~~~~~~~~~~~~~~~~~~~

## Rotisserie Chicken

1   precooked rotisserie chicken

Pick up from your favorite store and remove skin before eating. Serves 4.

**Serve with** ½ cup mashed potatoes, 1 cup Italian green beans and a 1-ounce dinner roll with 1 teaspoon reduced-fat margarine.

**Exchanges: 3 meats, 2 breads, 1 vegetable, 1 fat**

~~~~~~~~~~~~~~~~~~~~~~~~~~~~~~~~~~~~~~~~~~~~~~~~~~~

## Quick Baked Fish

1 ½   lbs. cod, tilapia, catfish or haddock fillets
¼   c. low-fat mayonnaise
1   tsp. Dijon mustard
2   tsp. dried onion flakes
1   tsp. white wine Worcestershire sauce
1   tsp. Old Bay seasoning
¼   tsp. paprika
1   tbsp. dried parsley
½   tsp. lemon pepper
⅛   tsp. cayenne pepper
Nonstick cooking spray

Preheat oven to 400° F. Wash fillets with cold water and pat dry with paper towels. Place fish fillets in a shallow casserole dish coated with nonstick cooking spray. In a small bowl, combine remaining ingredients; spread mixture evenly over fillets. Bake, uncovered, 15 minutes or until fish flakes easily with a fork. Serves 4.

**Serve with** steamed broccoli, ½ cup cooked brown rice and a 1-ounce bread stick.

**Exchanges: 3 meats, 2 breads, 1 vegetable, 1 fat**

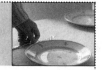

## Asparagus with Lemon Sauce

  1   10-oz. package frozen asparagus spears

  1   egg

       Sugar substitute to equal ½ cup sugar

 ½  tsp. cornstarch

  1   tbsp. margarine

 ¼  c. lemon juice

  2   tsp. grated lemon rind

Cook asparagus according to package directions, omitting salt and fat. Drain well. Transfer cooked asparagus to a serving dish and keep warm. Combine egg, sugar substitute and cornstarch. Melt margarine over low heat in a small skillet; add egg mixture. Cook over medium heat until mixture thickens. Stir in lemon juice. Continue to cook over medium heat until thickened and bubbly. Pour over asparagus; sprinkle with lemon rind. Serves 6.

**Exchange: 1 vegetable**

## Cheese Casserole Bread

  1   c. all-purpose flour

  1   c. whole-wheat flour

  1   tbsp. baking powder

  1   tbsp. dried minced onion

 ½  tsp. salt

       Sugar substitute to equal 2 tbsp. sugar

 ½  tsp. Italian herb seasoning

 ⅓  c. nonfat milk

 ¼  c. reduced-fat margarine, melted

  2   eggs, beaten

  1   tbsp. grated Parmesan cheese

       Nonstick cooking spray

Preheat oven to 400° F. In a medium bowl, combine flours, baking powder, onion, salt, sugar substitute and Italian herb seasoning; make a well in center of mixture. In a separate bowl, combine milk, margarine and eggs; add to dry ingredients, stirring just until moistened. Spoon batter into a round, 1 ½-quart casserole dish coated with non-stick cooking spray. Sprinkle with Parmesan cheese. Bake 25 to 30 minutes or until a wooden pick inserted in center comes out clean. Let stand 10 minutes; slice and serve warm, or turn out onto a wire rack and cool completely before slicing. Serves 12.

**Exchanges: 1 bread, 1 fat**

~~~~~~~~~~~~~~~~~~~~~~~~~~~~~~~~~~~~~~~~~~~~~~~~~~~~~~~~~~~~~~

## Creamed Potato Soup

4   medium red potatoes, peeled and cut into eighths
1   small onion, peeled and cut into eighths
4   green onions, coarsely chopped
1   clove garlic, minced
2   10 ½-oz. cans no-salt-added chicken broth
1   c. nonfat milk
½   tsp. salt
⅛   tsp. white pepper
⅛   tsp. nutmeg

Combine potatoes, onion, green onions, garlic and broth in a heavy 3-quart saucepan. Cover and simmer 20 minutes or until potatoes are tender. Blend potato mixture in an electric blender or food processor until smooth. Combine pureed mixture with milk, salt, pepper and nutmeg. Reheat soup to serving temperature or cover and refrigerate until thoroughly chilled. Serves 9.

**Exchanges: 1 bread**

~~~~~~~~~~~~~~~~~~~~~~~~~~~~~~~~~~~~~~~~~~~~~~~~~~~~~~~~~~~~~~

## Garden Vegetable Marinade

2   c. low-fat Italian dressing
    Sugar substitute to equal ¾ c. sugar
2   cloves garlic, minced
1   tsp. salt

Combine all ingredients in a jar. Cover tightly and shake vigorously. Store in refrigerator until ready to use as a marinade. Yields 2 cups marinade.

**Exchange: Free**

## Marinated Garden Vegetables

1 medium zucchini, sliced
1 medium cucumber, sliced
1 c. broccoli flowerets
2 c. cauliflower flowerets
2 c. sliced carrots
½ c. chopped green pepper
½ c. sliced celery
    *Garden Vegetable Marinade*
4 small tomatoes, quartered
1 c. sliced fresh mushrooms

Combine zucchini, cucumber, broccoli, cauliflower, carrots, green pepper and celery in a large bowl. Toss with *Garden Vegetable Marinade*; cover and refrigerate at least 12 hours, stirring occasionally. Add tomatoes and mushrooms just before serving. Makes 10 servings (1 cup each).

**Exchange: 1 vegetable**

## Mexican Cornbread

1 c. self-rising cornmeal
1 c. (4 oz.) shredded low-fat American cheese
1 c. whole-kernel corn
1 c. nonfat milk
½ c. chopped onion
1 4-oz. jar diced pimientos, drained
⅓ c. reduced-fat margarine
2 tbsp. chopped jalapeño peppers
½ tsp. garlic powder
    Nonstick cooking spray

Preheat oven to 350° F. Combine all ingredients, except nonstick cooking spray, in a large bowl and stir well. Pour batter into a 10½-inch cast-iron skillet coated with nonstick cooking spray. Bake 45 minutes or until golden brown; serve warm. Makes 10 squares.

**Exchanges: 1 bread, 1 fat**

## Parmesan Peas

2 10-oz. packages frozen peas
1 tbsp. grated Parmesan cheese
1 tsp. lemon juice
1 tsp. reduced-calorie margarine, melted
¼ tsp. Italian seasoning
⅛ tsp. grated lemon rind

Cook peas according to package directions, omitting salt and fat; drain. Toss peas with remaining ingredients and serve. Serves 6.

**Exchange: 1 vegetable**

## Sautéed Greens

1 medium onion, diced
1 tsp. olive oil
1 large bunch fresh greens (kale, collards, turnips or mustard greens), washed, cleaned and chopped (or 1 lb. frozen, thawed)
¼ c. vegetable broth
1 tbsp. balsamic vinegar

In a large skillet, sauté onion in olive oil over medium heat until tender. Add chopped greens, broth and vinegar; sauté 8 to 10 minutes more or until tender. Serves 4.

**Exchange: 1 vegetable**

## Peach Crumb Bake

2 c. sliced fresh peaches
⅓ c. graham cracker crumbs
½ tsp. ground cinnamon
⅛ tsp. ground nutmeg
2 tsp. margarine, melted
Nonstick cooking spray

Preheat oven to 350° F. Layer sliced peaches in bottom of an 8-inch square baking dish coated with nonstick cooking spray. In a small bowl, combine graham cracker crumbs, cinnamon and nutmeg. Add margarine; stir until crumbly. Sprinkle graham cracker crumb mixture over peaches. Bake 30 minutes. Serve warm. Makes 4 servings (½ cup each).
**Exchanges: 1 fruit, ½ fat**

~ ~ ~ ~ ~ ~ ~ ~ ~ ~ ~ ~ ~ ~ ~ ~ ~ ~ ~ ~ ~ ~ ~ ~ ~ ~ ~ ~ ~ ~ ~ ~ ~ ~ ~ ~ ~ ~ ~ ~ ~ ~ ~ ~ ~ ~ ~

## French Apple Tart

1 c. plus 1 tbsp. Grape Nuts cereal
⅓ c. plus 3 tbsp. apple juice concentrate, divided
½ tsp. cinnamon, divided
3 medium apples, peeled, cored and thinly sliced
2 tsp. lemon juice
1 tbsp. cornstarch
⅔ c. water

Preheat oven to 350°F. Moisten the cereal with 3 tbsp. apple juice concentrate in a 9 x 9-inch nonstick baking pan and pat into a thin layer. Sprinkle with ¼ teaspoon of cinnamon. Arrange the sliced apples over the cereal mixture in rows, overlapping slightly. Sprinkle with lemon juice and remaining ¼ teaspoon of cinnamon. Cover with aluminum foil. Bake 45 minutes or until apples are tender. Remove tart from oven and cool to room temperature. Combine cornstarch, remaining ⅓ cup apple juice concentrate and water in a saucepan. Cook over medium heat until mixture thickens and is clear, stirring constantly. Spoon mixture over the tart

or glaze with a pastry brush. Serve chilled or at room temperature. Serves 6.
**Exchanges: 1 bread, 1 fruit**

~~~~~~~~~~~~~~~~~~~~~~~~~~~~~~~~~~~~~~~~~~~~~~~~~~~~~~~~~~~

## *Fudge Candy*

     1   12-oz. can evaporated nonfat milk
     3   tbsp. cocoa
    ¼   c. reduced-fat margarine
    12   pkgs. sugar substitute, divided
         Dash salt
     5   c. puffed-rice cereal, crushed into crumbs
     1   tsp. vanilla extract
    ¼   c. nuts, finely chopped

Combine milk and cocoa in a saucepan; cook and whisk over low heat until cocoa is dissolved. Add margarine, 4 packages sugar substitute and salt. Bring to a boil; reduce heat and cook 5 minutes. Remove from heat; add cereal crumbs and vanilla. Cool 15 minutes. Add remaining 8 packages sugar substitute. Divide in half; roll each half into a tube shape and roll in finely chopped nuts. Wrap in waxed paper; chill overnight. Makes 32 slices.
**Exchanges for 2 slices: ½ bread, ½ fat**

# CONVERSION CHART
## EQUIVALENT IMPERIAL AND METRIC MEASUREMENTS

### Liquid Measures

| Fluid Ounces | U.S. | Imperial | Milliliters |
|---|---|---|---|
|  | 1 teaspoon | 1 teaspoon | 5 |
| $\frac{1}{4}$ | 2 teaspoons | 1 dessert spoon | 7 |
| $\frac{1}{2}$ | 1 tablespoon | 1 tablespoon | 15 |
| 1 | 2 tablespoons | 2 tablespoons | 28 |
| 2 | $\frac{1}{4}$ cup | 4 tablespoons | 56 |
| 4 | $\frac{1}{2}$ cup or $\frac{1}{4}$ pint |  | 110 |
| 5 |  | $\frac{1}{4}$ pint or 1 gill | 140 |
| 6 | $\frac{3}{4}$ cup |  | 170 |
| 8 | 1 cup or $\frac{1}{2}$ pint |  | 225 |
| 9 |  |  | 250 or $\frac{1}{4}$ liter |
| 10 | $1\frac{1}{4}$ cups | $\frac{1}{2}$ pint | 280 |
| 12 | $1\frac{1}{2}$ cups or $\frac{3}{4}$ pint |  | 340 |
| 15 |  | $\frac{3}{4}$ pint | 420 |
| 16 | 2 cups or 1 pint |  | 450 |
| 18 | $2\frac{1}{4}$ cups |  | 500 or $\frac{1}{2}$ liter |
| 20 | $2\frac{1}{2}$ cups | 1 pint | 560 |
| 24 | 3 cups or $1\frac{1}{2}$ pints |  | 675 |
| 25 |  | $1\frac{1}{4}$ pints | 700 |
| 30 | $3\frac{3}{4}$ cups | $1\frac{1}{2}$ pints | 840 |
| 32 | 4 cups |  | 900 |
| 36 | $4\frac{1}{2}$ cups |  | 1,000 or 1 liter |
| 40 | 5 cups | 2 pints or 1 quart | 1,120 |
| 48 | 6 cups or 3 pints |  | 1,350 |
| 50 |  | $2\frac{1}{2}$ pints | 1,400 |

## Solid Measures

| U.S. and Imperial Measures | | Metric Measures | |
|---|---|---|---|
| Ounces | Pounds | Grams | Kilos |
| 1 | | 28 | |
| 2 | | 56 | |
| $3\frac{1}{2}$ | | 100 | |
| 4 | $\frac{1}{4}$ | 112 | |
| 5 | | 140 | |
| 6 | | 168 | |
| 8 | $\frac{1}{2}$ | 225 | |
| 9 | | 250 | $\frac{1}{4}$ |
| 12 | $\frac{3}{4}$ | 340 | |
| 16 | 1 | 450 | |
| 18 | | 500 | $\frac{1}{2}$ |
| 20 | $1\frac{1}{4}$ | 560 | |
| 24 | | 675 | |
| 27 | | 750 | $\frac{3}{4}$ |
| 32 | 2 | 900 | |
| 36 | $2\frac{1}{4}$ | 1,000 | 1 |
| 40 | $2\frac{1}{2}$ | 1,100 | |
| 48 | 3 | 1,350 | |
| 54 | | 1,500 | $1\frac{1}{2}$ |
| 64 | 4 | 1,800 | |
| 72 | $4\frac{1}{2}$ | 2,000 | 2 |
| 80 | 5 | 2,250 | $2\frac{1}{4}$ |
| 100 | 6 | 2,800 | $2\frac{3}{4}$ |

# Oven Temperature Equivalents

| Fahrenheit | Celsius | Gas Mark | Description |
|---|---|---|---|
| 225 | 110 | ¼ | Cool |
| 250 | 130 | ½ | |
| 275 | 140 | 1 | Very Slow |
| 300 | 150 | 2 | |
| 325 | 170 | 3 | Slow |
| 350 | 180 | 4 | Moderate |
| 375 | 190 | 5 | |
| 400 | 200 | 6 | Moderately Hot |
| 425 | 220 | 7 | Fairly Hot |
| 450 | 230 | 8 | Hot |
| 475 | 240 | 9 | Very Hot |
| 500 | 250 | 10 | Extremely Hot |

# PERSONAL WEIGHT RECORD

| Week | Weight | + or - | Goal This Session | Pounds to Goal |
|------|--------|--------|-------------------|----------------|
| 1 | | | | |
| 2 | | | | |
| 3 | | | | |
| 4 | | | | |
| 5 | | | | |
| 6 | | | | |
| 7 | | | | |
| 8 | | | | |
| 9 | | | | |
| 10 | | | | |
| 11 | | | | |
| 12 | | | | |
| 13 | | | | |
| Final | | | | |

**Beginning Measurements**

Waist_____ Hips_____ Thighs_____ Chest_____

**Ending Measurements**

Waist_____ Hips_____ Thighs_____ Chest_____

# COMMITMENT RECORDS

## How to Fill Out a Commitment Record

The Commitment Record (CR) is an aid for you in keeping track of your accomplishments. Begin a new CR on the morning of the day your class meets. This ensures that your CR is complete before your next meeting. Turn in the CR weekly to your leader.

## FIRST PLACE CR

Name_____

Date_____through_____

Week # _____Calorie Level _____

Choose your calorie level.

### Daily Exchange Plan

| Level | Meat | Bread | Veggie | Fruit | Milk | Fat |
|-------|------|-------|--------|-------|------|-----|
| 1200  | 4-5  | 5-6   | 3      | 2-3   | 2-3  | 3-4 |
| 1400  | 5-6  | 6-7   | 3-4    | 3-4   | 2-3  | 3-4 |
| 1500  | 5-6  | 7-8   | 3-4    | 3-4   | 2-3  | 3-4 |
| 1600  | 6-7  | 8-9   | 3-4    | 3-4   | 2-3  | 3-4 |
| 1800  | 6-7  | 10-11 | 3-4    | 3-4   | 2-3  | 4-5 |
| 2000  | 6-7  | 11-12 | 4-5    | 4-5   | 2-3  | 4-5 |
| 2200  | 7-8  | 12-13 | 4-5    | 4-5   | 2-3  | 6-7 |
| 2400  | 8-9  | 13-14 | 4-5    | 4-5   | 2-3  | 7-8 |
| 2600  | 9-10 | 14-15 | 5      | 5     | 2-3  | 7-8 |
| 2800  | 9-10 | 15-16 | 5      | 5     | 2-3  | 9   |

Limit your high-range selections to only one of the following each day: meat, bread, milk or fat.

**Weekly Progress**

_____Loss _____Gain _____Maintain

At the end of each week, complete the weekly progress.

___ Attendance  ___ Bible Study
___ Prayer  ___ Scripture Reading
___ Memory Verse  ___ CR
___ Encouragement _____
___ Exercise:

Aerobic _____

_____

Strength _____

Flexibility _____

Record the number of days you kept the commitment.

Write the initials of the group member you encouraged this week.

## DAY 7:  Date _____

Morning _____
_____
_____

Midday _____
_____
_____

Evening _____
_____
_____

Snacks _____
_____
_____

___ Meat _____   ☐ Prayer
___ Bread _____   ☐ Bible Study
___ Vegetable _____   ☐ Scripture Reading
___ Fruit _____   ☐ Memory Verse
___ Milk _____   ☐ Encouragement
___ Fat _____   ☐ Water_____

**Exercise**

Aerobic _____
_____

Strength _____

Flexibility _____

List the foods you have eaten. On this condensed CR it is not necessary to exchange each food choice. It will be the responsibility of each member that the tally marks you list below are accurate regarding each food choice. If you are unsure of an exchange, check the Live-It section of your copy of the *Member's Guide*.

List the daily food exchange choices to the left of the food groups.

Use tally marks for the actual food and water consumed.

Check off commitments completed. Use tally marks to record each 8-oz. serving of water.

List type and duration of exercise.

# FIRST PLACE CR

Name _____

Date _____ through _____

Week # _____ Calorie Level _____

## Daily Exchange Plan

| Level | Meat | Bread | Veggie | Fruit | Milk | Fat |
|---|---|---|---|---|---|---|
| 1200 | 4-5 | 5-6 | 3 | 2-3 | 2-3 | 3-4 |
| 1400 | 5-6 | 6-7 | 3-4 | 3-4 | 2-3 | 3-4 |
| 1500 | 5-6 | 7-8 | 3-4 | 3-4 | 2-3 | 3-4 |
| 1600 | 6-7 | 8-9 | 3-4 | 3-4 | 2-3 | 3-4 |
| 1800 | 6-7 | 10-11 | 3-4 | 3-4 | 2-3 | 4-5 |
| 2000 | 6-7 | 11-12 | 4-5 | 4-5 | 2-3 | 4-5 |
| 2200 | 7-8 | 12-13 | 4-5 | 4-5 | 2-3 | 6-7 |
| 2400 | 8-9 | 13-14 | 4-5 | 4-5 | 2-3 | 7-8 |
| 2600 | 9-10 | 14-15 | 5 | 5 | 2-3 | 7-8 |
| 2800 | 9-10 | 15-16 | 5 | 5 | 2-3 | 9 |

You may always choose the high range of vegetables and fruits. Limit your high range selections to only one of the following: meat, bread, milk or fat.

## Weekly Progress

_____ Loss _____ Gain _____ Maintain

_____ Attendance _____ Bible Study
_____ Prayer _____ Scripture Reading
_____ Memory Verse _____ CR
_____ Encouragement:
_____ Exercise
Aerobic

Strength
Flexibility

---

## DAY 5: Date _____

Morning

Midday

Evening

Snacks

_____ Meat
_____ Bread
_____ Vegetable
_____ Fruit
_____ Milk
_____ Fat

☐ Prayer
☐ Bible Study
☐ Scripture Reading
☐ Memory Verse
☐ Encouragement
_____ Water

Exercise
Aerobic

Strength
Flexibility

---

## DAY 6: Date _____

Morning

Midday

Evening

Snacks

_____ Meat
_____ Bread
_____ Vegetable
_____ Fruit
_____ Milk
_____ Fat

☐ Prayer
☐ Bible Study
☐ Scripture Reading
☐ Memory Verse
☐ Encouragement
_____ Water

Exercise
Aerobic

Strength
Flexibility

---

## DAY 7: Date _____

Morning

Midday

Evening

Snacks

_____ Meat
_____ Bread
_____ Vegetable
_____ Fruit
_____ Milk
_____ Fat

☐ Prayer
☐ Bible Study
☐ Scripture Reading
☐ Memory Verse
☐ Encouragement
_____ Water

Exercise
Aerobic

Strength
Flexibility

# DAY 1: Date _____

Morning _____

Midday _____

Evening _____

Snacks _____

| Food | | Spiritual |
|---|---|---|
| ___ Meat | | ☐ Prayer |
| ___ Bread | | ☐ Bible Study |
| ___ Vegetable | | ☐ Scripture Reading |
| ___ Fruit | | ☐ Memory Verse |
| ___ Milk | | ☐ Encouragement |
| ___ Fat | ___ Water | |

Exercise
Aerobic _____
Strength _____
Flexibility _____

# DAY 2: Date _____

Morning _____

Midday _____

Evening _____

Snacks _____

| Food | | Spiritual |
|---|---|---|
| ___ Meat | | ☐ Prayer |
| ___ Bread | | ☐ Bible Study |
| ___ Vegetable | | ☐ Scripture Reading |
| ___ Fruit | | ☐ Memory Verse |
| ___ Milk | | ☐ Encouragement |
| ___ Fat | ___ Water | |

Exercise
Aerobic _____
Strength _____
Flexibility _____

# DAY 3: Date _____

Morning _____

Midday _____

Evening _____

Snacks _____

| Food | | Spiritual |
|---|---|---|
| ___ Meat | | ☐ Prayer |
| ___ Bread | | ☐ Bible Study |
| ___ Vegetable | | ☐ Scripture Reading |
| ___ Fruit | | ☐ Memory Verse |
| ___ Milk | | ☐ Encouragement |
| ___ Fat | ___ Water | |

Exercise
Aerobic _____
Strength _____
Flexibility _____

# DAY 4: Date _____

Morning _____

Midday _____

Evening _____

Snacks _____

| Food | | Spiritual |
|---|---|---|
| ___ Meat | | ☐ Prayer |
| ___ Bread | | ☐ Bible Study |
| ___ Vegetable | | ☐ Scripture Reading |
| ___ Fruit | | ☐ Memory Verse |
| ___ Milk | | ☐ Encouragement |
| ___ Fat | ___ Water | |

Exercise
Aerobic _____
Strength _____
Flexibility _____

# FIRST PLACE CR

Name _____
Date _____ through _____
Week # _____ Calorie Level _____

### Daily Exchange Plan

| Level | Meat | Bread | Veggie | Fruit | Milk | Fat |
|---|---|---|---|---|---|---|
| 1200 | 4-5 | 5-6 | 3 | 2-3 | 2-3 | 3-4 |
| 1400 | 5-6 | 6-7 | 3-4 | 3-4 | 2-3 | 3-4 |
| 1500 | 5-6 | 7-8 | 3-4 | 3-4 | 2-3 | 3-4 |
| 1600 | 6-7 | 8-9 | 3-4 | 3-4 | 2-3 | 3-4 |
| 1800 | 6-7 | 10-11 | 3-4 | 3-4 | 2-3 | 4-5 |
| 2000 | 6-7 | 11-12 | 4-5 | 4-5 | 2-3 | 4-5 |
| 2200 | 7-8 | 12-13 | 4-5 | 4-5 | 2-3 | 6-7 |
| 2400 | 8-9 | 13-14 | 4-5 | 4-5 | 2-3 | 7-8 |
| 2600 | 9-10 | 14-15 | 5 | 5 | 2-3 | 7-8 |
| 2800 | 9-10 | 15-16 | 5 | 5 | 2-3 | 9 |

You may always choose the high range of vegetables and fruits. Limit your high range selections to only one of the following: meat, bread, milk or fat.

**Weekly Progress**

_____ Loss _____ Gain _____ Maintain

_____ Attendance _____ Bible Study
_____ Prayer _____ Scripture Reading
_____ Memory Verse _____ CR
_____ Encouragement:
_____ Exercise
Aerobic _____
Strength _____
Flexibility _____

---

## DAY 5: Date _____

Morning _____

Midday _____

Evening _____

Snacks _____

_____ Meat ☐ Prayer
_____ Bread ☐ Bible Study
_____ Vegetable ☐ Scripture Reading
_____ Fruit ☐ Memory Verse
_____ Milk ☐ Encouragement
_____ Fat _____ Water
Exercise
Aerobic _____

Strength _____
Flexibility _____

---

## DAY 6: Date _____

Morning _____

Midday _____

Evening _____

Snacks _____

_____ Meat ☐ Prayer
_____ Bread ☐ Bible Study
_____ Vegetable ☐ Scripture Reading
_____ Fruit ☐ Memory Verse
_____ Milk ☐ Encouragement
_____ Fat _____ Water
Exercise
Aerobic _____

Strength _____
Flexibility _____

---

## DAY 7: Date _____

Morning _____

Midday _____

Evening _____

Snacks _____

_____ Meat ☐ Prayer
_____ Bread ☐ Bible Study
_____ Vegetable ☐ Scripture Reading
_____ Fruit ☐ Memory Verse
_____ Milk ☐ Encouragement
_____ Fat _____ Water
Exercise
Aerobic _____

Strength _____
Flexibility _____

## DAY 1: Date _____

Morning _____

Midday _____

Evening _____

Snacks _____

| | |
|---|---|
| ___ Meat | ☐ Prayer |
| ___ Bread | ☐ Bible Study |
| ___ Vegetable | ☐ Scripture Reading |
| ___ Fruit | ☐ Memory Verse |
| ___ Milk | ☐ Encouragement |
| ___ Fat ___ Water | |

**Exercise**
Aerobic _____
Strength _____
Flexibility _____

## DAY 2: Date _____

Morning _____

Midday _____

Evening _____

Snacks _____

| | |
|---|---|
| ___ Meat | ☐ Prayer |
| ___ Bread | ☐ Bible Study |
| ___ Vegetable | ☐ Scripture Reading |
| ___ Fruit | ☐ Memory Verse |
| ___ Milk | ☐ Encouragement |
| ___ Fat ___ Water | |

**Exercise**
Aerobic _____
Strength _____
Flexibility _____

## DAY 3: Date _____

Morning _____

Midday _____

Evening _____

Snacks _____

| | |
|---|---|
| ___ Meat | ☐ Prayer |
| ___ Bread | ☐ Bible Study |
| ___ Vegetable | ☐ Scripture Reading |
| ___ Fruit | ☐ Memory Verse |
| ___ Milk | ☐ Encouragement |
| ___ Fat ___ Water | |

**Exercise**
Aerobic _____
Strength _____
Flexibility _____

## DAY 4: Date _____

Morning _____

Midday _____

Evening _____

Snacks _____

| | |
|---|---|
| ___ Meat | ☐ Prayer |
| ___ Bread | ☐ Bible Study |
| ___ Vegetable | ☐ Scripture Reading |
| ___ Fruit | ☐ Memory Verse |
| ___ Milk | ☐ Encouragement |
| ___ Fat ___ Water | |

**Exercise**
Aerobic _____
Strength _____
Flexibility _____

Name _____

Date _____ through _____

Week # _____ Calorie Level _____

### Daily Exchange Plan

| Level | Meat | Bread | Veggie | Fruit | Milk | Fat |
|---|---|---|---|---|---|---|
| 1200 | 4-5 | 5-6 | 3 | 2-3 | 2-3 | 3-4 |
| 1400 | 5-6 | 6-7 | 3-4 | 3-4 | 2-3 | 3-4 |
| 1500 | 5-6 | 7-8 | 3-4 | 3-4 | 2-3 | 3-4 |
| 1600 | 6-7 | 8-9 | 3-4 | 3-4 | 2-3 | 3-4 |
| 1800 | 6-7 | 10-11 | 3-4 | 3-4 | 2-3 | 4-5 |
| 2000 | 6-7 | 11-12 | 4-5 | 4-5 | 2-3 | 4-5 |
| 2200 | 7-8 | 12-13 | 4-5 | 4-5 | 2-3 | 6-7 |
| 2400 | 8-9 | 13-14 | 4-5 | 4-5 | 2-3 | 6-7 |
| 2600 | 9-10 | 14-15 | 5 | 5 | 2-3 | 7-8 |
| 2800 | 9-10 | 15-16 | 5 | 5 | 2-3 | 9 |

You may always choose the high range of vegetables and fruits. Limit your high range selections to only one of the following: meat, bread, milk or fat.

**Weekly Progress**

____ Loss ____ Gain ____ Maintain

____ Attendance ____ Bible Study
____ Prayer ____ Scripture Reading
____ Memory Verse ____ CR
____ Encouragement:
____ Exercise
Aerobic _____
Strength _____
Flexibility _____

---

## DAY 5: Date _____

Morning _____

Midday _____

Evening _____

Snacks _____

____ Meat _____  ☐ Prayer
____ Bread _____  ☐ Bible Study
____ Vegetable ____  ☐ Scripture Reading
____ Fruit _____  ☐ Memory Verse
____ Milk _____   ☐ Encouragement
____ Fat _____    Water ____
**Exercise**
Aerobic _____
Strength _____
Flexibility _____

---

## DAY 6: Date _____

Morning _____

Midday _____

Evening _____

Snacks _____

____ Meat _____  ☐ Prayer
____ Bread _____  ☐ Bible Study
____ Vegetable ____  ☐ Scripture Reading
____ Fruit _____  ☐ Memory Verse
____ Milk _____   ☐ Encouragement
____ Fat _____    Water ____
**Exercise**
Aerobic _____
Strength _____
Flexibility _____

---

## DAY 7: Date _____

Morning _____

Midday _____

Evening _____

Snacks _____

____ Meat _____  ☐ Prayer
____ Bread _____  ☐ Bible Study
____ Vegetable ____  ☐ Scripture Reading
____ Fruit _____  ☐ Memory Verse
____ Milk _____   ☐ Encouragement
____ Fat _____    Water ____
**Exercise**
Aerobic _____
Strength _____
Flexibility _____

## DAY 1: Date _____

Morning _____

Midday _____

Evening _____

Snacks _____

| | |
|---|---|
| ___ Meat | ☐ Prayer |
| ___ Bread | ☐ Bible Study |
| ___ Vegetable | ☐ Scripture Reading |
| ___ Fruit | ☐ Memory Verse |
| ___ Milk | ☐ Encouragement |
| ___ Fat | ___ Water |

**Exercise**
Aerobic _____
Strength _____
Flexibility _____

## DAY 2: Date _____

Morning _____

Midday _____

Evening _____

Snacks _____

| | |
|---|---|
| ___ Meat | ☐ Prayer |
| ___ Bread | ☐ Bible Study |
| ___ Vegetable | ☐ Scripture Reading |
| ___ Fruit | ☐ Memory Verse |
| ___ Milk | ☐ Encouragement |
| ___ Fat | ___ Water |

**Exercise**
Aerobic _____
Strength _____
Flexibility _____

## DAY 3: Date _____

Morning _____

Midday _____

Evening _____

Snacks _____

| | |
|---|---|
| ___ Meat | ☐ Prayer |
| ___ Bread | ☐ Bible Study |
| ___ Vegetable | ☐ Scripture Reading |
| ___ Fruit | ☐ Memory Verse |
| ___ Milk | ☐ Encouragement |
| ___ Fat | ___ Water |

**Exercise**
Aerobic _____
Strength _____
Flexibility _____

## DAY 4: Date _____

Morning _____

Midday _____

Evening _____

Snacks _____

| | |
|---|---|
| ___ Meat | ☐ Prayer |
| ___ Bread | ☐ Bible Study |
| ___ Vegetable | ☐ Scripture Reading |
| ___ Fruit | ☐ Memory Verse |
| ___ Milk | ☐ Encouragement |
| ___ Fat | ___ Water |

**Exercise**
Aerobic _____
Strength _____
Flexibility _____

# FIRST PLACE CR

Name _____

Date _____ through _____

Week # _____ Calorie Level _____

## Daily Exchange Plan

| Level | Meat | Bread | Veggie | Fruit | Milk | Fat |
|---|---|---|---|---|---|---|
| 1200 | 4-5 | 5-6 | 3 | 2-3 | 2-3 | 3-4 |
| 1400 | 5-6 | 6-7 | 3-4 | 3-4 | 2-3 | 3-4 |
| 1500 | 5-6 | 7-8 | 3-4 | 3-4 | 2-3 | 3-4 |
| 1600 | 6-7 | 8-9 | 3-4 | 3-4 | 2-3 | 3-4 |
| 1800 | 6-7 | 10-11 | 3-4 | 3-4 | 2-3 | 4-5 |
| 2000 | 6-7 | 11-12 | 4-5 | 4-5 | 2-3 | 4-5 |
| 2200 | 7-8 | 12-13 | 4-5 | 4-5 | 2-3 | 6-7 |
| 2400 | 8-9 | 13-14 | 4-5 | 4-5 | 2-3 | 7-8 |
| 2600 | 9-10 | 14-15 | 5 | 5 | 2-3 | 7-8 |
| 2800 | 9-10 | 15-16 | 5 | 5 | 2-3 | 9 |

You may always choose the high range of vegetables and fruits. Limit your high range selections to only one of the following: meat, bread, milk or fat.

### Weekly Progress

_____ Loss _____ Gain _____ Maintain

_____ Attendance _____ Bible Study
_____ Prayer _____ Scripture Reading
_____ Memory Verse _____ CR
_____ Encouragement:
_____ Exercise
Aerobic _____
Strength _____
Flexibility _____

---

## DAY 5: Date _____

Morning _____

Midday _____

Evening _____

Snacks _____

_____ Meat       ☐ Prayer
_____ Bread      ☐ Bible Study
_____ Vegetable  ☐ Scripture Reading
_____ Fruit      ☐ Memory Verse
_____ Milk       ☐ Encouragement
_____ Fat        Water _____
Exercise
Aerobic _____
Strength _____
Flexibility _____

## DAY 6: Date _____

Morning _____

Midday _____

Evening _____

Snacks _____

_____ Meat       ☐ Prayer
_____ Bread      ☐ Bible Study
_____ Vegetable  ☐ Scripture Reading
_____ Fruit      ☐ Memory Verse
_____ Milk       ☐ Encouragement
_____ Fat        Water _____
Exercise
Aerobic _____
Strength _____
Flexibility _____

## DAY 7: Date _____

Morning _____

Midday _____

Evening _____

Snacks _____

_____ Meat       ☐ Prayer
_____ Bread      ☐ Bible Study
_____ Vegetable  ☐ Scripture Reading
_____ Fruit      ☐ Memory Verse
_____ Milk       ☐ Encouragement
_____ Fat        Water _____
Exercise
Aerobic _____
Strength _____
Flexibility _____

## DAY 1: Date _____

Morning _____

Midday _____

Evening _____

Snacks _____

| | |
|---|---|
| ___ Meat | ☐ Prayer |
| ___ Bread | ☐ Bible Study |
| ___ Vegetable | ☐ Scripture Reading |
| ___ Fruit | ☐ Memory Verse |
| ___ Milk | ☐ Encouragement |
| ___ Fat | ___ Water |

**Exercise**
Aerobic _____
Strength _____
Flexibility _____

## DAY 2: Date _____

Morning _____

Midday _____

Evening _____

Snacks _____

| | |
|---|---|
| ___ Meat | ☐ Prayer |
| ___ Bread | ☐ Bible Study |
| ___ Vegetable | ☐ Scripture Reading |
| ___ Fruit | ☐ Memory Verse |
| ___ Milk | ☐ Encouragement |
| ___ Fat | ___ Water |

**Exercise**
Aerobic _____
Strength _____
Flexibility _____

## DAY 3: Date _____

Morning _____

Midday _____

Evening _____

Snacks _____

| | |
|---|---|
| ___ Meat | ☐ Prayer |
| ___ Bread | ☐ Bible Study |
| ___ Vegetable | ☐ Scripture Reading |
| ___ Fruit | ☐ Memory Verse |
| ___ Milk | ☐ Encouragement |
| ___ Fat | ___ Water |

**Exercise**
Aerobic _____
Strength _____
Flexibility _____

## DAY 4: Date _____

Morning _____

Midday _____

Evening _____

Snacks _____

| | |
|---|---|
| ___ Meat | ☐ Prayer |
| ___ Bread | ☐ Bible Study |
| ___ Vegetable | ☐ Scripture Reading |
| ___ Fruit | ☐ Memory Verse |
| ___ Milk | ☐ Encouragement |
| ___ Fat | ___ Water |

**Exercise**
Aerobic _____
Strength _____
Flexibility _____

# FIRST PLACE CR

Name _____

Date _____ through _____

Week # _____  Calorie Level _____

## Daily Exchange Plan

| Level | Meat | Bread | Veggie | Fruit | Milk | Fat |
|-------|------|-------|--------|-------|------|-----|
| 1200 | 4-5 | 5-6 | 3 | 2-3 | 2-3 | 3-4 |
| 1400 | 5-6 | 6-7 | 3-4 | 3-4 | 2-3 | 3-4 |
| 1500 | 5-6 | 7-8 | 3-4 | 3-4 | 2-3 | 3-4 |
| 1600 | 6-7 | 8-9 | 3-4 | 3-4 | 2-3 | 3-4 |
| 1800 | 6-7 | 10-11 | 3-4 | 3-4 | 2-3 | 4-5 |
| 2000 | 6-7 | 11-12 | 4-5 | 4-5 | 2-3 | 4-5 |
| 2200 | 7-8 | 12-13 | 4-5 | 4-5 | 2-3 | 6-7 |
| 2400 | 8-9 | 13-14 | 4-5 | 4-5 | 2-3 | 7-8 |
| 2600 | 9-10 | 14-15 | 5 | 5 | 2-3 | 7-8 |
| 2800 | 9-10 | 15-16 | 5 | 5 | 2-3 | 9 |

You may always choose the high range of vegetables and fruits. Limit your high range selections to only one of the following: meat, bread, milk or fat.

### Weekly Progress

_____ Loss _____ Gain _____ Maintain

_____ Attendance _____ Bible Study

_____ Prayer _____ Scripture Reading

_____ Memory Verse _____ CR

_____ Encouragement: _____

_____ Exercise

Aerobic _____

Strength _____

Flexibility _____

---

## DAY 5: Date _____

Morning _____

Midday _____

Evening _____

Snacks _____

_____ Meat          ☐ Prayer
_____ Bread         ☐ Bible Study
_____ Vegetable     ☐ Scripture Reading
_____ Fruit         ☐ Memory Verse
_____ Milk          ☐ Encouragement
_____ Fat           _____ Water

Exercise
Aerobic _____

Strength _____
Flexibility _____

---

## DAY 6: Date _____

Morning _____

Midday _____

Evening _____

Snacks _____

_____ Meat          ☐ Prayer
_____ Bread         ☐ Bible Study
_____ Vegetable     ☐ Scripture Reading
_____ Fruit         ☐ Memory Verse
_____ Milk          ☐ Encouragement
_____ Fat           _____ Water

Exercise
Aerobic _____

Strength _____
Flexibility _____

---

## DAY 7: Date _____

Morning _____

Midday _____

Evening _____

Snacks _____

_____ Meat          ☐ Prayer
_____ Bread         ☐ Bible Study
_____ Vegetable     ☐ Scripture Reading
_____ Fruit         ☐ Memory Verse
_____ Milk          ☐ Encouragement
_____ Fat           _____ Water

Exercise
Aerobic _____

Strength _____
Flexibility _____

## DAY 1: Date_____

Morning _____

Midday _____

Evening _____

Snacks _____

| | |
|---|---|
| ___ Meat | ☐ Prayer |
| ___ Bread | ☐ Bible Study |
| ___ Vegetable | ☐ Scripture Reading |
| ___ Fruit | ☐ Memory Verse |
| ___ Milk | ☐ Encouragement |
| ___ Fat | ___ Water |

**Exercise**
Aerobic _____
Strength _____
Flexibility _____

## DAY 2: Date_____

Morning _____

Midday _____

Evening _____

Snacks _____

| | |
|---|---|
| ___ Meat | ☐ Prayer |
| ___ Bread | ☐ Bible Study |
| ___ Vegetable | ☐ Scripture Reading |
| ___ Fruit | ☐ Memory Verse |
| ___ Milk | ☐ Encouragement |
| ___ Fat | ___ Water |

**Exercise**
Aerobic _____
Strength _____
Flexibility _____

## DAY 3: Date_____

Morning _____

Midday _____

Evening _____

Snacks _____

| | |
|---|---|
| ___ Meat | ☐ Prayer |
| ___ Bread | ☐ Bible Study |
| ___ Vegetable | ☐ Scripture Reading |
| ___ Fruit | ☐ Memory Verse |
| ___ Milk | ☐ Encouragement |
| ___ Fat | ___ Water |

**Exercise**
Aerobic _____
Strength _____
Flexibility _____

## DAY 4: Date_____

Morning _____

Midday _____

Evening _____

Snacks _____

| | |
|---|---|
| ___ Meat | ☐ Prayer |
| ___ Bread | ☐ Bible Study |
| ___ Vegetable | ☐ Scripture Reading |
| ___ Fruit | ☐ Memory Verse |
| ___ Milk | ☐ Encouragement |
| ___ Fat | ___ Water |

**Exercise**
Aerobic _____
Strength _____
Flexibility _____

# FIRST PLACE CR

Name _____

Date _____ through _____

Week # _____ Calorie Level _____

## Daily Exchange Plan

| Level | Meat | Bread | Veggie | Fruit | Milk | Fat |
|---|---|---|---|---|---|---|
| 1200 | 4-5 | 5-6 | 3 | 2-3 | 2-3 | 3-4 |
| 1400 | 5-6 | 6-7 | 3-4 | 3-4 | 2-3 | 3-4 |
| 1500 | 5-6 | 7-8 | 3-4 | 3-4 | 2-3 | 3-4 |
| 1600 | 6-7 | 8-9 | 3-4 | 3-4 | 2-3 | 3-4 |
| 1800 | 6-7 | 10-11 | 3-4 | 3-4 | 2-3 | 4-5 |
| 2000 | 6-7 | 11-12 | 4-5 | 4-5 | 2-3 | 4-5 |
| 2200 | 7-8 | 12-13 | 4-5 | 4-5 | 2-3 | 6-7 |
| 2400 | 8-9 | 13-14 | 4-5 | 4-5 | 2-3 | 7-8 |
| 2600 | 9-10 | 14-15 | 5 | 5 | 2-3 | 7-8 |
| 2800 | 9-10 | 15-16 | 5 | 5 | 2-3 | 9 |

You may always choose the high range of vegetables and fruits. Limit your high range selections to only one of the following: meat, bread, milk or fat.

## Weekly Progress

_____ Loss  _____ Gain  _____ Maintain

_____ Attendance  _____ Bible Study
_____ Prayer  _____ Scripture Reading
_____ Memory Verse  _____ CR
_____ Encouragement:
_____ Exercise
_____ Aerobic

_____ Strength
_____ Flexibility

---

## DAY 5: Date _____

Morning _____

Midday _____

Evening _____

Snacks _____

_____ Meat        ☐ Prayer
_____ Bread       ☐ Bible Study
_____ Vegetable   ☐ Scripture Reading
_____ Fruit       ☐ Memory Verse
_____ Milk        ☐ Encouragement
_____ Fat         _____ Water

Exercise
Aerobic _____

Strength _____
Flexibility _____

---

## DAY 6: Date _____

Morning _____

Midday _____

Evening _____

Snacks _____

_____ Meat        ☐ Prayer
_____ Bread       ☐ Bible Study
_____ Vegetable   ☐ Scripture Reading
_____ Fruit       ☐ Memory Verse
_____ Milk        ☐ Encouragement
_____ Fat         _____ Water

Exercise
Aerobic _____

Strength _____
Flexibility _____

---

## DAY 7: Date _____

Morning _____

Midday _____

Evening _____

Snacks _____

_____ Meat        ☐ Prayer
_____ Bread       ☐ Bible Study
_____ Vegetable   ☐ Scripture Reading
_____ Fruit       ☐ Memory Verse
_____ Milk        ☐ Encouragement
_____ Fat         _____ Water

Exercise
Aerobic _____

Strength _____
Flexibility _____

## DAY 1:  Date _____

Morning _____

Midday _____

Evening _____

Snacks _____

| | |
|---|---|
| ___ Meat | ☐ Prayer |
| ___ Bread | ☐ Bible Study |
| ___ Vegetable | ☐ Scripture Reading |
| ___ Fruit | ☐ Memory Verse |
| ___ Milk | ☐ Encouragement |
| ___ Fat | ___ Water |

Exercise
Aerobic _____
Strength _____
Flexibility _____

## DAY 2:  Date _____

Morning _____

Midday _____

Evening _____

Snacks _____

| | |
|---|---|
| ___ Meat | ☐ Prayer |
| ___ Bread | ☐ ...ble Study |
| ___ Vegetable | ☐ Scripture Reading |
| ___ Fruit | ☐ Memory Verse |
| ___ Milk | ☐ Encouragement |
| ___ Fat | ___ Water |

Exercise
Aerobic _____
Strength _____
Flexibility _____

## DAY 3:  Date _____

Morning _____

Midday _____

Evening _____

Snacks _____

| | |
|---|---|
| ___ Meat | ☐ Prayer |
| ___ Bread | ☐ Bible Study |
| ___ Vegetable | ☐ Scripture Reading |
| ___ Fruit | ☐ Memory Verse |
| ___ Milk | ☐ Encouragement |
| ___ Fat | ___ Water |

Exercise
Aerobic _____
Strength _____
Flexibility _____

## DAY 4:  Date _____

Morning _____

Midday _____

Evening _____

Snacks _____

| | |
|---|---|
| ___ Meat | ☐ Prayer |
| ___ Bread | ☐ Bible Study |
| ___ Vegetable | ☐ Scripture Reading |
| ___ Fruit | ☐ Memory Verse |
| ___ Milk | ☐ Encouragement |
| ___ Fat | ___ Water |

Exercise
Aerobic _____
Strength _____
Flexibility _____

# FIRST PLACE CR

Name _____

Date _____ through _____
Week # _____ Calorie Level _____

## Daily Exchange Plan

| Level | Meat | Bread | Veggie | Fruit | Milk | Fat |
|-------|------|-------|--------|-------|------|-----|
| 1200 | 4-5 | 5-6 | 3 | 2-3 | 2-3 | 3-4 |
| 1400 | 5-6 | 6-7 | 3-4 | 3-4 | 2-3 | 3-4 |
| 1500 | 5-6 | 7-8 | 3-4 | 3-4 | 2-3 | 3-4 |
| 1600 | 6-7 | 8-9 | 3-4 | 3-4 | 2-3 | 3-4 |
| 1800 | 6-7 | 10-11 | 3-4 | 3-4 | 2-3 | 4-5 |
| 2000 | 6-7 | 11-12 | 4-5 | 4-5 | 2-3 | 4-5 |
| 2200 | 7-8 | 12-13 | 4-5 | 4-5 | 2-3 | 6-7 |
| 2400 | 8-9 | 13-14 | 4-5 | 4-5 | 2-3 | 7-8 |
| 2600 | 9-10 | 14-15 | 5 | 5 | 2-3 | 7-8 |
| 2800 | 9-10 | 15-16 | 5 | 5 | 2-3 | 9 |

You may always choose the high range of vegetables and fruits. Limit your high range selections to only one of the following: meat, bread, milk or fat.

### Weekly Progress

_____ Loss _____ Gain _____ Maintain

_____ Attendance      _____ Bible Study
_____ Prayer          _____ Scripture Reading
_____ Memory Verse    _____ CR
_____ Encouragement:
_____ Exercise
Aerobic _____

Strength _____
Flexibility _____

---

## DAY 5: Date _____

Morning _____

Midday _____

Evening _____

Snacks _____

_____ Meat          ☐ Prayer
_____ Bread         ☐ Bible Study
_____ Vegetable     ☐ Scripture Reading
_____ Fruit         ☐ Memory Verse
_____ Milk          ☐ Encouragement
_____ Fat           ☐ Water

Exercise
Aerobic _____

Strength _____
Flexibility _____

---

## DAY 6: Date _____

Morning _____

Midday _____

Evening _____

Snacks _____

_____ Meat          ☐ Prayer
_____ Bread         ☐ Bible Study
_____ Vegetable     ☐ Scripture Reading
_____ Fruit         ☐ Memory Verse
_____ Milk          ☐ Encouragement
_____ Fat           ☐ Water

Exercise
Aerobic _____

Strength _____
Flexibility _____

---

## DAY 7: Date _____

Morning _____

Midday _____

Evening _____

Snacks _____

_____ Meat          ☐ Prayer
_____ Bread         ☐ Bible Study
_____ Vegetable     ☐ Scripture Reading
_____ Fruit         ☐ Memory Verse
_____ Milk          ☐ Encouragement
_____ Fat           ☐ Water

Exercise
Aerobic _____

Strength _____
Flexibility _____

## DAY 1: Date _____

**Morning** _____

**Midday** _____

**Evening** _____

**Snacks** _____

| | |
|---|---|
| ___ **Meat** ___ | ☐ Prayer |
| ___ **Bread** ___ | ☐ Bible Study |
| ___ **Vegetable** ___ | ☐ Scripture Reading |
| ___ **Fruit** ___ | ☐ Memory Verse |
| ___ **Milk** ___ | ☐ Encouragement |
| ___ **Fat** ___ | ___ Water ___ |

**Exercise**
Aerobic _____
Strength _____
Flexibility _____

## DAY 2: Date _____

**Morning** _____

**Midday** _____

**Evening** _____

**Snacks** _____

| | |
|---|---|
| ___ **Meat** ___ | ☐ Prayer |
| ___ **Bread** ___ | ☐ Bible Study |
| ___ **Vegetable** ___ | ☐ Scripture Reading |
| ___ **Fruit** ___ | ☐ Memory Verse |
| ___ **Milk** ___ | ☐ Encouragement |
| ___ **Fat** ___ | ___ Water ___ |

**Exercise**
Aerobic _____
Strength _____
Flexibility _____

## DAY 3: Date _____

**Morning** _____

**Midday** _____

**Evening** _____

**Snacks** _____

| | |
|---|---|
| ___ **Meat** ___ | ☐ Prayer |
| ___ **Bread** ___ | ☐ Bible Study |
| ___ **Vegetable** ___ | ☐ Scripture Reading |
| ___ **Fruit** ___ | ☐ Memory Verse |
| ___ **Milk** ___ | ☐ Encouragement |
| ___ **Fat** ___ | ___ Water ___ |

**Exercise**
Aerobic _____
Strength _____
Flexibility _____

## DAY 4: Date _____

**Morning** _____

**Midday** _____

**Evening** _____

**Snacks** _____

| | |
|---|---|
| ___ **Meat** ___ | ☐ Prayer |
| ___ **Bread** ___ | ☐ Bible Study |
| ___ **Vegetable** ___ | ☐ Scripture Reading |
| ___ **Fruit** ___ | ☐ Memory Verse |
| ___ **Milk** ___ | ☐ Encouragement |
| ___ **Fat** ___ | ___ Water ___ |

**Exercise**
Aerobic _____
Strength _____
Flexibility _____

# FIRST PLACE CR

Name _____

Date _____ through _____

Week # _____ Calorie Level _____

## Daily Exchange Plan

| Level | Meat | Bread | Veggie | Fruit | Milk | Fat |
|-------|------|-------|--------|-------|------|-----|
| 1200 | 4-5 | 5-6 | 3 | 2-3 | 2-3 | 3-4 |
| 1400 | 5-6 | 6-7 | 3-4 | 3-4 | 2-3 | 3-4 |
| 1500 | 5-6 | 7-8 | 3-4 | 3-4 | 2-3 | 3-4 |
| 1600 | 6-7 | 8-9 | 3-4 | 3-4 | 2-3 | 3-4 |
| 1800 | 6-7 | 10-11 | 3-4 | 3-4 | 2-3 | 4-5 |
| 2000 | 6-7 | 11-12 | 4-5 | 4-5 | 2-3 | 4-5 |
| 2200 | 7-8 | 12-13 | 4-5 | 4-5 | 2-3 | 6-7 |
| 2400 | 8-9 | 13-14 | 4-5 | 4-5 | 2-3 | 7-8 |
| 2600 | 9-10 | 14-15 | 5 | 5 | 2-3 | 7-8 |
| 2800 | 9-10 | 15-16 | 5 | 5 | 2-3 | 9 |

You may always choose the high range of vegetables and fruits. Limit your high range selections to only one of the following: meat, bread, milk or fat.

## Weekly Progress

_____ Loss _____ Gain _____ Maintain

_____ Attendance _____ Bible Study
_____ Prayer _____ Scripture Reading
_____ Memory Verse _____ CR
_____ Encouragement:
_____ Exercise
_____ Aerobic

Strength _____
Flexibility _____

---

## DAY 5: Date _____

Morning _____

Midday _____

Evening _____

Snacks _____

_____ Meat        ☐ Prayer
_____ Bread       ☐ Bible Study
_____ Vegetable   ☐ Scripture Reading
_____ Fruit       ☐ Memory Verse
_____ Milk        ☐ Encouragement
_____ Fat         _____ Water

Exercise
Aerobic _____

Strength _____
Flexibility _____

---

## DAY 6: Date _____

Morning _____

Midday _____

Evening _____

Snacks _____

_____ Meat        ☐ Prayer
_____ Bread       ☐ Bible Study
_____ Vegetable   ☐ Scripture Reading
_____ Fruit       ☐ Memory Verse
_____ Milk        ☐ Encouragement
_____ Fat         _____ Water

Exercise
Aerobic _____

Strength _____
Flexibility _____

---

## DAY 7: Date _____

Morning _____

Midday _____

Evening _____

Snacks _____

_____ Meat        ☐ Prayer
_____ Bread       ☐ Bible Study
_____ Vegetable   ☐ Scripture Reading
_____ Fruit       ☐ Memory Verse
_____ Milk        ☐ Encouragement
_____ Fat         _____ Water

Exercise
Aerobic _____

Strength _____
Flexibility _____

# DAY 1: Date _____

Morning _____

Midday _____

Evening _____

Snacks _____

| Meat _____ | ☐ Prayer |
| Bread _____ | ☐ Bible Study |
| Vegetable _____ | ☐ Scripture Reading |
| Fruit _____ | ☐ Memory Verse |
| Milk _____ | ☐ Encouragement |
| Fat _____ | Water _____ |

**Exercise**
Aerobic _____
Strength _____
Flexibility _____

# DAY 2: Date _____

Morning _____

Midday _____

Evening _____

Snacks _____

| Meat _____ | ☐ Prayer |
| Bread _____ | ☐ Bible Study |
| Vegetable _____ | ☐ Scripture Reading |
| Fruit _____ | ☐ Memory Verse |
| Milk _____ | ☐ Encouragement |
| Fat _____ | Water _____ |

**Exercise**
Aerobic _____
Strength _____
Flexibility _____

# DAY 3: Date _____

Morning _____

Midday _____

Evening _____

Snacks _____

| Meat _____ | ☐ Prayer |
| Bread _____ | ☐ Bible Study |
| Vegetable _____ | ☐ Scripture Reading |
| Fruit _____ | ☐ Memory Verse |
| Milk _____ | ☐ Encouragement |
| Fat _____ | Water _____ |

**Exercise**
Aerobic _____
Strength _____
Flexibility _____

# DAY 4: Date _____

Morning _____

Midday _____

Evening _____

Snacks _____

| Meat _____ | ☐ Prayer |
| Bread _____ | ☐ Bible Study |
| Vegetable _____ | ☐ Scripture Reading |
| Fruit _____ | ☐ Memory Verse |
| Milk _____ | ☐ Encouragement |
| Fat _____ | Water _____ |

**Exercise**
Aerobic _____
Strength _____
Flexibility _____

# FIRST PLACE CR

Name _____

Date _____ through _____

Week # _____ Calorie Level _____

## Daily Exchange Plan

| Level | Meat | Bread | Veggie | Fruit | Milk | Fat |
|-------|------|-------|--------|-------|------|-----|
| 1200 | 4-5 | 5-6 | 3 | 2-3 | 2-3 | 3-4 |
| 1400 | 5-6 | 6-7 | 3-4 | 3-4 | 2-3 | 3-4 |
| 1500 | 5-6 | 7-8 | 3-4 | 3-4 | 2-3 | 3-4 |
| 1600 | 6-7 | 8-9 | 3-4 | 3-4 | 2-3 | 3-4 |
| 1800 | 6-7 | 10-11 | 3-4 | 3-4 | 2-3 | 4-5 |
| 2000 | 6-7 | 11-12 | 4-5 | 4-5 | 2-3 | 4-5 |
| 2200 | 7-8 | 12-13 | 4-5 | 4-5 | 2-3 | 6-7 |
| 2400 | 8-9 | 13-14 | 4-5 | 4-5 | 2-3 | 7-8 |
| 2600 | 9-10 | 14-15 | 5 | 5 | 2-3 | 7-8 |
| 2800 | 9-10 | 15-16 | 5 | 5 | 2-3 | 9 |

You may always choose the high range of vegetables and fruits. Limit your high range selections to only one of the following: meat, bread, milk or fat.

### Weekly Progress

___ Loss ___ Gain ___ Maintain

___ Attendance ___ Bible Study
___ Prayer ___ Scripture Reading
___ Memory Verse ___ CR
___ Encouragement:
___ Exercise
Aerobic _____
Strength _____
Flexibility _____

---

## DAY 7: Date _____

Morning _____

Midday _____

Evening _____

Snacks _____

___ Meat ☐ Prayer
___ Bread ☐ Bible Study
___ Vegetable ☐ Scripture Reading
___ Fruit ☐ Memory Verse
___ Milk ☐ Encouragement
___ Fat ___ Water

Exercise
Aerobic _____
Strength _____
Flexibility _____

---

## DAY 6: Date _____

Morning _____

Midday _____

Evening _____

Snacks _____

___ Meat ☐ Prayer
___ Bread ☐ Bible Study
___ Vegetable ☐ Scripture Reading
___ Fruit ☐ Memory Verse
___ Milk ☐ Encouragement
___ Fat ___ Water

Exercise
Aerobic _____
Strength _____
Flexibility _____

---

## DAY 5: Date _____

Morning _____

Midday _____

Evening _____

Snacks _____

___ Meat ☐ Prayer
___ Bread ☐ Bible Study
___ Vegetable ☐ Scripture Reading
___ Fruit ☐ Memory Verse
___ Milk ☐ Encouragement
___ Fat ___ Water

Exercise
Aerobic _____
Strength _____
Flexibility _____

## DAY 1: Date _____

Morning _____

Midday _____

Evening _____

Snacks _____

| Meat _____ | ☐ Prayer |
| Bread _____ | ☐ Bible Study |
| Vegetable _____ | ☐ Scripture Reading |
| Fruit _____ | ☐ Memory Verse |
| Milk _____ | ☐ Encouragement |
| Fat _____ | Water _____ |

**Exercise**
Aerobic _____
Strength _____
Flexibility _____

## DAY 2: Date _____

Morning _____

Midday _____

Evening _____

Snacks _____

| Meat _____ | ☐ Prayer |
| Bread _____ | ☐ Bible Study |
| Vegetable _____ | ☐ Scripture Reading |
| Fruit _____ | ☐ Memory Verse |
| Milk _____ | ☐ Encouragement |
| Fat _____ | Water _____ |

**Exercise**
Aerobic _____
Strength _____
Flexibility _____

## DAY 3: Date _____

Morning _____

Midday _____

Evening _____

Snacks _____

| Meat _____ | ☐ Prayer |
| Bread _____ | ☐ Bible Study |
| Vegetable _____ | ☐ Scripture Reading |
| Fruit _____ | ☐ Memory Verse |
| Milk _____ | ☐ Encouragement |
| Fat _____ | Water _____ |

**Exercise**
Aerobic _____
Strength _____
Flexibility _____

## DAY 4: Date _____

Morning _____

Midday _____

Evening _____

Snacks _____

| Meat _____ | ☐ Prayer |
| Bread _____ | ☐ Bible Study |
| Vegetable _____ | ☐ Scripture Reading |
| Fruit _____ | ☐ Memory Verse |
| Milk _____ | ☐ Encouragement |
| Fat _____ | Water _____ |

**Exercise**
Aerobic _____
Strength _____
Flexibility _____

# FIRST PLACE CR

Name _____

Date _____ through _____

Week # _____ Calorie Level _____

## Daily Exchange Plan

| Level | Meat | Bread | Veggie | Fruit | Milk | Fat |
|-------|------|-------|--------|-------|------|-----|
| 1200 | 4-5 | 5-6 | 3 | 2-3 | 2-3 | 3-4 |
| 1400 | 5-6 | 6-7 | 3-4 | 3-4 | 2-3 | 3-4 |
| 1500 | 5-6 | 7-8 | 3-4 | 3-4 | 2-3 | 3-4 |
| 1600 | 6-7 | 8-9 | 3-4 | 3-4 | 2-3 | 3-4 |
| 1800 | 6-7 | 10-11 | 3-4 | 3-4 | 2-3 | 4-5 |
| 2000 | 6-7 | 11-12 | 4-5 | 4-5 | 2-3 | 4-5 |
| 2200 | 7-8 | 12-13 | 4-5 | 4-5 | 2-3 | 6-7 |
| 2400 | 8-9 | 13-14 | 4-5 | 4-5 | 2-3 | 7-8 |
| 2600 | 9-10 | 14-15 | 5 | 5 | 2-3 | 7-8 |
| 2800 | 9-10 | 15-16 | 5 | 5 | 2-3 | 9 |

You may always choose the high range of vegetables and fruits. Limit your high range selections to only one of the following: meat, bread, milk or fat.

## Weekly Progress

_____ Loss _____ Gain _____ Maintain

_____ Attendance _____ Bible Study

_____ Prayer _____ Scripture Reading

_____ Memory Verse _____ CR

_____ Encouragement: _____

_____ Exercise _____

Aerobic _____

Strength _____

Flexibility _____

---

## DAY 7: Date _____

Morning _____

Midday _____

Evening _____

Snacks _____

_____ Meat ☐ Prayer
_____ Bread ☐ Bible Study
_____ Vegetable ☐ Scripture Reading
_____ Fruit ☐ Memory Verse
_____ Milk ☐ Encouragement
_____ Fat _____ Water

Exercise
Aerobic _____

Strength _____
Flexibility _____

---

## DAY 6: Date _____

Morning _____

Midday _____

Evening _____

Snacks _____

_____ Meat ☐ Prayer
_____ Bread ☐ Bible Study
_____ Vegetable ☐ Scripture Reading
_____ Fruit ☐ Memory Verse
_____ Milk ☐ Encouragement
_____ Fat _____ Water

Exercise
Aerobic _____

Strength _____
Flexibility _____

---

## DAY 5: Date _____

Morning _____

Midday _____

Evening _____

Snacks _____

_____ Meat ☐ Prayer
_____ Bread ☐ Bible Study
_____ Vegetable ☐ Scripture Reading
_____ Fruit ☐ Memory Verse
_____ Milk ☐ Encouragement
_____ Fat _____ Water

Exercise
Aerobic _____

Strength _____
Flexibility _____

## DAY 1: Date _____

Morning _____

Midday _____

Evening _____

Snacks _____

| | | |
|---|---|---|
| ___ Meat ___ | ☐ Prayer |
| ___ Bread ___ | ☐ Bible Study |
| ___ Vegetable ___ | ☐ Scripture Reading |
| ___ Fruit ___ | ☐ Memory Verse |
| ___ Milk ___ | ☐ Encouragement |
| ___ Fat ___ Water ___ | |

**Exercise**
Aerobic _____
Strength _____
Flexibility _____

## DAY 2: Date _____

Morning _____

Midday _____

Evening _____

Snacks _____

| | | |
|---|---|---|
| ___ Meat ___ | ☐ Prayer |
| ___ Bread ___ | ☐ Bible Study |
| ___ Vegetable ___ | ☐ Scripture Reading |
| ___ Fruit ___ | ☐ Memory Verse |
| ___ Milk ___ | ☐ Encouragement |
| ___ Fat ___ Water ___ | |

**Exercise**
Aerobic _____
Strength _____
Flexibility _____

## DAY 3: Date _____

Morning _____

Midday _____

Evening _____

Snacks _____

| | | |
|---|---|---|
| ___ Meat ___ | ☐ Prayer |
| ___ Bread ___ | ☐ Bible Study |
| ___ Vegetable ___ | ☐ Scripture Reading |
| ___ Fruit ___ | ☐ Memory Verse |
| ___ Milk ___ | ☐ Encouragement |
| ___ Fat ___ Water ___ | |

**Exercise**
Aerobic _____
Strength _____
Flexibility _____

## DAY 4: Date _____

Morning _____

Midday _____

Evening _____

Snacks _____

| | | |
|---|---|---|
| ___ Meat ___ | ☐ Prayer |
| ___ Bread ___ | ☐ Bible Study |
| ___ Vegetable ___ | ☐ Scripture Reading |
| ___ Fruit ___ | ☐ Memory Verse |
| ___ Milk ___ | ☐ Encouragement |
| ___ Fat ___ Water ___ | |

**Exercise**
Aerobic _____
Strength _____
Flexibility _____

# FIRST PLACE CR

Name _____
Date _____ through _____
Week # _____ Calorie Level _____

## Daily Exchange Plan

| Level | Meat | Bread | Veggie | Fruit | Milk | Fat |
|---|---|---|---|---|---|---|
| 1200 | 4-5 | 5-6 | 3 | 2-3 | 2-3 | 3-4 |
| 1400 | 5-6 | 6-7 | 3-4 | 3-4 | 2-3 | 3-4 |
| 1500 | 5-6 | 7-8 | 3-4 | 3-4 | 2-3 | 3-4 |
| 1600 | 6-7 | 8-9 | 3-4 | 3-4 | 2-3 | 3-4 |
| 1800 | 6-7 | 10-11 | 3-4 | 3-4 | 2-3 | 4-5 |
| 2000 | 6-7 | 11-12 | 4-5 | 4-5 | 2-3 | 4-5 |
| 2200 | 7-8 | 12-13 | 4-5 | 4-5 | 2-3 | 6-7 |
| 2400 | 8-9 | 13-14 | 4-5 | 4-5 | 2-3 | 7-8 |
| 2600 | 9-10 | 14-15 | 5 | 5 | 2-3 | 7-8 |
| 2800 | 9-10 | 15-16 | 5 | 5 | 2-3 | 9 |

You may always choose the high range of vegetables and fruits. Limit your high range selections to only one of the following: meat, bread, milk or fat.

### Weekly Progress

Loss _____ Gain _____ Maintain _____

___ Attendance   ___ Bible Study
___ Prayer        ___ Scripture Reading
___ Memory Verse  ___ CR
___ Encouragement:
___ Exercise
Aerobic _____
Strength _____
Flexibility _____

---

## DAY 5: Date _____

Morning _____

Midday _____

Evening _____

Snacks _____

___ Meat
___ Bread
___ Vegetable
___ Fruit
___ Milk
___ Fat
___ Water

☐ Prayer
☐ Bible Study
☐ Scripture Reading
☐ Memory Verse
☐ Encouragement

Exercise
Aerobic _____
Strength _____
Flexibility _____

---

## DAY 6: Date _____

Morning _____

Midday _____

Evening _____

Snacks _____

___ Meat
___ Bread
___ Vegetable
___ Fruit
___ Milk
___ Fat
___ Water

☐ Prayer
☐ Bible Study
☐ Scripture Reading
☐ Memory Verse
☐ Encouragement

Exercise
Aerobic _____
Strength _____
Flexibility _____

---

## DAY 7: Date _____

Morning _____

Midday _____

Evening _____

Snacks _____

___ Meat
___ Bread
___ Vegetable
___ Fruit
___ Milk
___ Fat
___ Water

☐ Prayer
☐ Bible Study
☐ Scripture Reading
☐ Memory Verse
☐ Encouragement

Exercise
Aerobic _____
Strength _____
Flexibility _____

## DAY 1: Date _____

Morning _____

Midday _____

Evening _____

Snacks _____

_____ Meat _____   ☐ Prayer
_____ Bread _____   ☐ Bible Study
_____ Vegetable _____   ☐ Scripture Reading
_____ Fruit _____   ☐ Memory Verse
_____ Milk _____   ☐ Encouragement
_____ Fat _____ Water _____

**Exercise**
Aerobic _____
Strength _____
Flexibility _____

## DAY 2: Date _____

Morning _____

Midday _____

Evening _____

Snacks _____

_____ Meat _____   ☐ Prayer
_____ Bread _____   ☐ Bible Study
_____ Vegetable _____   ☐ Scripture Reading
_____ Fruit _____   ☐ Memory Verse
_____ Milk _____   ☐ Encouragement
_____ Fat _____ Water _____

**Exercise**
Aerobic _____
Strength _____
Flexibility _____

## DAY 3: Date _____

Morning _____

Midday _____

Evening _____

Snacks _____

_____ Meat _____   ☐ Prayer
_____ Bread _____   ☐ Bible Study
_____ Vegetable _____   ☐ Scripture Reading
_____ Fruit _____   ☐ Memory Verse
_____ Milk _____   ☐ Encouragement
_____ Fat _____ Water _____

**Exercise**
Aerobic _____
Strength _____
Flexibility _____

## DAY 4: Date _____

Morning _____

Midday _____

Evening _____

Snacks _____

_____ Meat _____   ☐ Prayer
_____ Bread _____   ☐ Bible Study
_____ Vegetable _____   ☐ Scripture Reading
_____ Fruit _____   ☐ Memory Verse
_____ Milk _____   ☐ Encouragement
_____ Fat _____ Water _____

**Exercise**
Aerobic _____
Strength _____
Flexibility _____

# FIRST PLACE CR

Name _____

Date _____ through _____

Week # _____ Calorie Level _____

### Daily Exchange Plan

| Level | Meat | Bread | Veggie | Fruit | Milk | Fat |
|---|---|---|---|---|---|---|
| 1200 | 4-5 | 5-6 | 3 | 2-3 | 2-3 | 3-4 |
| 1400 | 5-6 | 6-7 | 3-4 | 3-4 | 2-3 | 3-4 |
| 1500 | 5-6 | 7-8 | 3-4 | 3-4 | 2-3 | 3-4 |
| 1600 | 6-7 | 8-9 | 3-4 | 3-4 | 2-3 | 3-4 |
| 1800 | 6-7 | 10-11 | 3-4 | 3-4 | 2-3 | 4-5 |
| 2000 | 6-7 | 11-12 | 4-5 | 4-5 | 2-3 | 4-5 |
| 2200 | 7-8 | 12-13 | 4-5 | 4-5 | 2-3 | 6-7 |
| 2400 | 8-9 | 13-14 | 4-5 | 4-5 | 2-3 | 7-8 |
| 2600 | 9-10 | 14-15 | 5 | 5 | 2-3 | 7-8 |
| 2800 | 9-10 | 15-16 | 5 | 5 | 2-3 | 9 |

You may always choose the high range of vegetables and fruits. Limit your high range selections to only one of the following: meat, bread, milk or fat.

### Weekly Progress

____ Loss ____ Gain ____ Maintain

____ Attendance ____ Bible Study
____ Prayer ____ Scripture Reading
____ Memory Verse ____ CR
____ Encouragement:
____ Exercise
Aerobic _____
Strength _____
Flexibility _____

---

## DAY 5: Date _____

Morning _____

Midday _____

Evening _____

Snacks _____

____ Meat    ☐ Prayer
____ Bread   ☐ Bible Study
____ Vegetable   ☐ Scripture Reading
____ Fruit   ☐ Memory Verse
____ Milk   ☐ Encouragement
____ Fat    Water _____

Exercise
Aerobic _____

Strength _____
Flexibility _____

---

## DAY 6: Date _____

Morning _____

Midday _____

Evening _____

Snacks _____

____ Meat    ☐ Prayer
____ Bread   ☐ Bible Study
____ Vegetable   ☐ Scripture Reading
____ Fruit   ☐ Memory Verse
____ Milk   ☐ Encouragement
____ Fat    Water _____

Exercise
Aerobic _____

Strength _____
Flexibility _____

---

## DAY 7: Date _____

Morning _____

Midday _____

Evening _____

Snacks _____

____ Meat    ☐ Prayer
____ Bread   ☐ Bible Study
____ Vegetable   ☐ Scripture Reading
____ Fruit   ☐ Memory Verse
____ Milk   ☐ Encouragement
____ Fat    Water _____

Exercise
Aerobic _____

Strength _____
Flexibility _____

## DAY 1: Date _____

Morning _____

Midday _____

Evening _____

Snacks _____

| ___ Meat | ☐ Prayer |
| ___ Bread | ☐ Bible Study |
| ___ Vegetable | ☐ Scripture Reading |
| ___ Fruit | ☐ Memory Verse |
| ___ Milk | ☐ Encouragement |
| ___ Fat | ___ Water |

**Exercise**

Aerobic _____

Strength _____

Flexibility _____

## DAY 2: Date _____

Morning _____

Midday _____

Evening _____

Snacks _____

| ___ Meat | ☐ Prayer |
| ___ Bread | ☐ Bible Study |
| ___ Vegetable | ☐ Scripture Reading |
| ___ Fruit | ☐ Memory Verse |
| ___ Milk | ☐ Encouragement |
| ___ Fat | ___ Water |

**Exercise**

Aerobic _____

Strength _____

Flexibility _____

## DAY 3: Date _____

Morning _____

Midday _____

Evening _____

Snacks _____

| ___ Meat | ☐ Prayer |
| ___ Bread | ☐ Bible Study |
| ___ Vegetable | ☐ Scripture Reading |
| ___ Fruit | ☐ Memory Verse |
| ___ Milk | ☐ Encouragement |
| ___ Fat | ___ Water |

**Exercise**

Aerobic _____

Strength _____

Flexibility _____

## DAY 4: Date _____

Morning _____

Midday _____

Evening _____

Snacks _____

| ___ Meat | ☐ Prayer |
| ___ Bread | ☐ Bible Study |
| ___ Vegetable | ☐ Scripture Reading |
| ___ Fruit | ☐ Memory Verse |
| ___ Milk | ☐ Encouragement |
| ___ Fat | ___ Water |

**Exercise**

Aerobic _____

Strength _____

Flexibility _____

# FIRST PLACE CR

Name _____

Date _____ through _____

Week # _____ Calorie Level _____

## Daily Exchange Plan

| Level | Meat | Bread | Veggie | Fruit | Milk | Fat |
|---|---|---|---|---|---|---|
| 1200 | 4-5 | 5-6 | 3 | 2-3 | 2-3 | 3-4 |
| 1400 | 5-6 | 6-7 | 3-4 | 3-4 | 2-3 | 3-4 |
| 1500 | 5-6 | 7-8 | 3-4 | 3-4 | 2-3 | 3-4 |
| 1600 | 6-7 | 8-9 | 3-4 | 3-4 | 2-3 | 3-4 |
| 1800 | 6-7 | 10-11 | 3-4 | 3-4 | 2-3 | 4-5 |
| 2000 | 6-7 | 11-12 | 4-5 | 4-5 | 2-3 | 4-5 |
| 2200 | 7-8 | 12-13 | 4-5 | 4-5 | 2-3 | 6-7 |
| 2400 | 8-9 | 13-14 | 4-5 | 4-5 | 2-3 | 7-8 |
| 2600 | 9-10 | 14-15 | 5 | 5 | 2-3 | 7-8 |
| 2800 | 9-10 | 15-16 | 5 | 5 | 2-3 | 9 |

You may always choose the high range of vegetables and fruits. Limit your high range selections to only one of the following: meat, bread, milk or fat.

### Weekly Progress

_____ Loss _____ Gain _____ Maintain

_____ Attendance _____ Bible Study
_____ Prayer _____ Scripture Reading
_____ Memory Verse _____ CR
_____ Encouragement:
_____ Exercise
Aerobic

Strength
Flexibility

---

## DAY 5: Date _____

Morning _____

Midday _____

Evening _____

Snacks _____

_____ Meat
_____ Bread
_____ Vegetable
_____ Fruit
_____ Milk
_____ Fat
Exercise
Aerobic _____

Strength _____
Flexibility _____

☐ Prayer
☐ Bible Study
☐ Scripture Reading
☐ Memory Verse
☐ Encouragement
☐ Water _____

---

## DAY 6: Date _____

Morning _____

Midday _____

Evening _____

Snacks _____

_____ Meat
_____ Bread
_____ Vegetable
_____ Fruit
_____ Milk
_____ Fat
Exercise
Aerobic _____

Strength _____
Flexibility _____

☐ Prayer
☐ Bible Study
☐ Scripture Reading
☐ Memory Verse
☐ Encouragement
☐ Water _____

---

## DAY 7: Date _____

Morning _____

Midday _____

Evening _____

Snacks _____

_____ Meat
_____ Bread
_____ Vegetable
_____ Fruit
_____ Milk
_____ Fat
Exercise
Aerobic _____

Strength _____
Flexibility _____

☐ Prayer
☐ Bible Study
☐ Scripture Reading
☐ Memory Verse
☐ Encouragement
☐ Water _____

# DAY 1: Date _____

Morning _____

Midday _____

Evening _____

Snacks _____

| | |
|---|---|
| ___ Meat | ☐ Prayer |
| ___ Bread | ☐ Bible Study |
| ___ Vegetable | ☐ Scripture Reading |
| ___ Fruit | ☐ Memory Verse |
| ___ Milk | ☐ Encouragement |
| ___ Fat | ___ Water |

Exercise
Aerobic _____
Strength _____
Flexibility _____

# DAY 2: Date _____

Morning _____

Midday _____

Evening _____

Snacks _____

| | |
|---|---|
| ___ Meat | ☐ Prayer |
| ___ Bread | ☐ Bible Study |
| ___ Vegetable | ☐ Scripture Reading |
| ___ Fruit | ☐ Memory Verse |
| ___ Milk | ☐ Encouragement |
| ___ Fat | ___ Water |

Exercise
Aerobic _____
Strength _____
Flexibility _____

# DAY 3: Date _____

Morning _____

Midday _____

Evening _____

Snacks _____

| | |
|---|---|
| ___ Meat | ☐ Prayer |
| ___ Bread | ☐ Bible Study |
| ___ Vegetable | ☐ Scripture Reading |
| ___ Fruit | ☐ Memory Verse |
| ___ Milk | ☐ Encouragement |
| ___ Fat | ___ Water |

Exercise
Aerobic _____
Strength _____
Flexibility _____

# DAY 4: Date _____

Morning _____

Midday _____

Evening _____

Snacks _____

| | |
|---|---|
| ___ Meat | ☐ Prayer |
| ___ Bread | ☐ Bible Study |
| ___ Vegetable | ☐ Scripture Reading |
| ___ Fruit | ☐ Memory Verse |
| ___ Milk | ☐ Encouragement |
| ___ Fat | ___ Water |

Exercise
Aerobic _____
Strength _____
Flexibility _____

# CONTRIBUTOR

**Elizabeth Crews** has a master's degree in Counseling/Psychology/ Family Systems Theory and is a licensed drug and alcohol counselor and educator. For 15 years, Elizabeth taught small groups and adult Sunday School classes while also serving as an elder for adult education in her local church. Currently, she leads a First Place group and is a networking leader.

# SCRIPTURE MEMORY VERSES

## Week One

Give thanks to the LORD, for he is good. His love endures forever (Psalm 136:1).

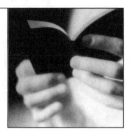

## Week Two

For the Mighty One has done great things for me—holy is his name (Luke 1:49).

## Week Three

He brought me out into a spacious place; he rescued me because he delighted in me (Psalm 18:19).

## Week Four

The Counselor, the Holy Spirit, whom the Father will send in my name, will teach you all things and will remind you of everything I have said to you (John 14:26).

## Week Five

What other nation is so great as to have their gods near them the way the LORD our God is near us whenever we pray to him (Deuteronomy 4:7)?

## Week Six

You, O LORD, keep my lamp burning; my God turns my darkness into light (Psalm 18:28).

## Week Seven

I rejoice in following your statutes as one rejoices in great riches (Psalm 119:14).

## Week Eight

He who did not spare his own Son, but gave him up for us all—how will he not also, along with him, graciously give us all things (Romans 8:32)?

## Week Nine

Therefore, since we are receiving a kingdom that cannot be shaken, let us be thankful, and so worship God acceptably with reverence and awe (Hebrews 12:28).

## Week Ten

Always giving thanks to God the Father for everything, in the name of our Lord Jesus Christ (Ephesians 5:20).

# Don't Miss the Companion Book to the *Choosing Thankfulness* Bible Study

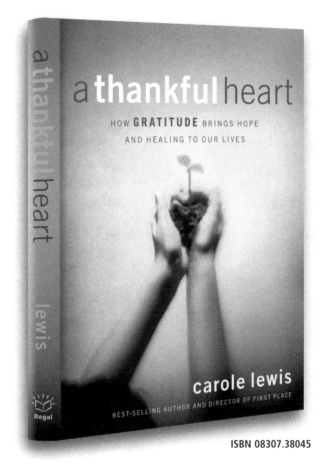

ISBN 08307.38045

## A Thankful Heart
### How Gratitude Brings Hope and Healing to Our Lives

Thankfulness is not a popular topic in today's world where complaining or criticizing is more the norm. More difficult still is being thankful in the midst of very challenging circumstances. In *A Thankful Heart*, Carole Lewis shares her personal experience of adopting a heart of gratitude after the untimely death of her daughter and how this act became a powerful tool of healing in her life. Citing other real-life examples of giving thanks, Carole shows how life is made up of moments, each one an opportunity to make the choice to give thanks.

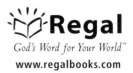

# Bible Studies to Help You Put Christ First

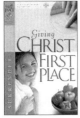

**Giving Christ
First Place**
Bible Study
*ISBN 08307.28643*

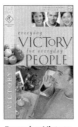

**Everyday Victory
for Everyday People**
Bible Study
*ISBN 08307.28651*

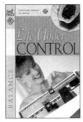

**Life Under Control**
Bible Study
*ISBN 08307.29305*

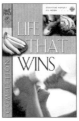

**Life That Wins**
Bible Study
*ISBN 08307.29240*

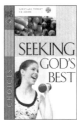

**Seeking God's Best**
Bible Study
*ISBN 08307.29259*

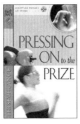

**Pressing On
to the Prize**
Bible Study
*ISBN 08307.29267*

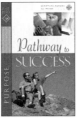

**Pathway to Success**
Bible Study
*ISBN 08307.29275*

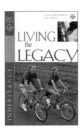

**Living the Legacy**
Bible Study
*ISBN 08307.29283*

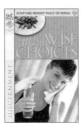

**Making Wise
Choices**
Bible Study
*ISBN 08307.30818*

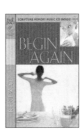

**Begin Again**
Bible Study
*ISBN 08307.32330*

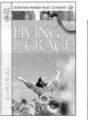

**Living in Grace**
Bible Study
*ISBN 08307.32349*

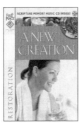

**A New Creation**
Bible Study
*ISBN 08307.33566*

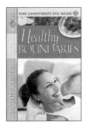

**Healthy Boundaries**
Bible Study
*ISBN 08307.38002*

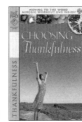

**Choosing Thankfulness**
Bible Study
*ISBN 08307.38185*

**FIRST PLACE™**

Available at bookstores everywhere or by calling
1-800-4-GOSPEL. **Join the First Place community
and order products at www.firstplace.org.**

**Gospel Light**

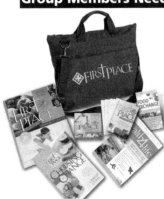